The Marlowe Diabetes Library
Good control is in your hands.

SINCE 1999, Marlowe & Company has established itself as the nation's leading independent publisher of books on diabetes. Now, the Marlowe Diabetes Library, launched in 2007, comprises an ever-expanding list of books on how to thrive while living with diabetes or prediabetes. Authors include world-renowned authorities on diabetes and the glycemic index, medical doctors and research scientists, certified diabetes educators, registered dietitians and other professional clinicians, as well as individuals living and thriving with prediabetes, type 1 or type 2 diabetes. See page 197 for the complete list of Marlowe Diabetes Library titles.

Diabetes on Your Own Terms

JANIS ROSZLER, RD, CDE, LD/N, is a registered dietitian, certified diabetes educator, insulin pump trainer, author, and radio host. She is the author of the popular "Dear Janis" column in *Diabetes Positive* magazine, monthly columnist for dLife.com, and contributor to numerous publications including *Diabetes Forecast, Diabetes Health,* and *Diabetes Self-Management* magazines. She was the host of *Janis' Jump Start to Good Health* on WWNN radio and is currently the host of the *dTalk Radio Show* on dLife.com. Janis travels internationally as a speaker on diabetes and other health-related topics and lives in Miami Beach, Florida, with her husband and four children.

ALSO BY
Janis Roszler
(with William H. Polonsky and Steven V. Edelman)

•

The Secrets of Living and Loving with Diabetes

DIABETES ON YOUR OWN TERMS

JANIS ROSZLER,
RD, CDE, LD/N

MARLOWE & COMPANY
NEW YORK

DIABETES ON YOUR OWN TERMS

Copyright © 2007 by Janis Roszler

Published by
Marlowe & Company
An Imprint of Avalon Publishing Group, Incorporated
245 West 17th Street • 11th Floor
New York, NY 10011–5300

AVALON

All rights reserved. No part of this book may be reproduced in whole or in part without written permission from the publisher, except by reviewers who may quote brief excerpts in connection with a review in a newspaper, magazine, or electronic publication; nor may any part of this book be reproduced, stored in a retrieval system, or transmitted in any form or by any means electronic, mechanical, photocopying, recording, or other, without written permission from the publisher.

The excerpt on page 106 from *Forbidden Foods Diabetic Cooking*, copyright © 2000 American Diabetes Association, is reprinted with permission from *The American Diabetes Association*.

Library of Congress Cataloging-in-Publication Data is available

ISBN-10: 1–56924–304–2
ISBN-13: 978–1–56924–304–6

9 8 7 6 5 4 3 2 1

Designed by Pauline Neuwirth, Neuwirth & Associates, Inc.

Printed in the United States of America

The information in this book is intended to help readers make informed decisions about their health and the health of their loved ones. It is not intended to be a substitute for treatment by or the advice and care of a professional health-care provider. While the author and publisher have endeavored to ensure that the information presented is accurate and up to date, they are not responsible for adverse effects or consequences sustained by any person using this book.

To my parents, Bob and Maxine Cohn,
who encouraged me to live life on my own terms.

Contents

INTRODUCTION	xv
1 SAY YES TO . . . Guilt Free Diabetes Control	1
STEP 1: *Evaluate Your Diabetes Control*	2
STEP 2: *Set Your Personal Blood Glucose Range*	8
2 SAY YES TO . . . Choosing the Right Medication Options	23
STEP 3: *Review Your Medication Options*	24
STEP 4: *Set Your A-B-C Goals*	43
3 SAY YES TO . . . Realistic Weight Goals	45
STEP 5: *Set Your Weight Goal*	46
STEP 6: *Choose the Right Meal-Planning Method for You*	53
4 SAY YES TO . . . A Life with Few or No Diabetes Complications	67
STEP 7: *Learn about Possible Complications*	68
STEP 8: *Choose Treatments that Will Work for You*	68
5 SAY YES TO . . . Getting the Guidance You Need	87
STEP 9: *Check Your Information*	88
STEP 10: *Be a Partner in Your Diabetes Care*	95

6 SAY YES TO ... Enjoying the Foods You Love   103
　STEP 11: *Examine Why You Desire Certain Foods*   104
　STEP 12: *Shop Wisely*   115

7 SAY YES TO ... An Active Social Life   119
　STEP 13: *Plan Ahead When You Socialize*   120
　STEP 14: *Prepare for Intimacy*   132

8 SAY YES TO ... A Less Stressful Life   137
　STEP 15: *Reduce the Stress in Your Life*   138
　STEP 16: *Seek Help for Depression, If Needed*   149

9 SAY YES TO ... Roads Well (and Less) Traveled   153
　STEP 17: *Don't Let Diabetes Stop You*   154
　STEP 18: *Expect the Unexpected*   157

10 SAY YES TO ... Changing the Future   165
　STEP 19: *Find a Way to Make a Difference*   167
　STEP 20: *Enjoy the Benefits of Helping Others*   176

AFTERWORD   179
SELECTED REFERENCES   181
RECOMMENDED BOOKS AND WEB SITES   183
ACKNOWLEDGMENTS   187
INDEX   189

Introduction

AT THE AGE of twenty, Kris Freeman was busy preparing for the 2002 Winter Olympics. He was a top U.S. cross-country skier with a promising career ahead of him. When he was suddenly diagnosed with type 1 diabetes, his world changed. He was told by several physicians that his skiing career was over—that it was not possible to have diabetes and compete at an elite level in an endurance sport. But Kris refused to accept that. He decided from the very start to find a way to create a personalized diabetes plan. And he did it. He assembled a supportive team of medical experts who suggested different approaches to blood glucose control and ultimately helped him develop a program that worked for him. He continued skiing and became a four-time national champion, the top cross-country skier in the United States, and a member of the United States 2006 Winter Olympics team. Says Kris:

> My advice is to learn as much as you can about the disease, to learn as much as you can about the treatments, to learn as much as you can about diet and what diets will work for you, to help you achieve whatever dream that you have.

Be prepared: this book may surprise you. I'm not going to offer you another miracle plan for perfect diabetes control—"one size fits all" methods rarely fit anyone. Instead, I'd like to open up a world of choices for you to explore. Like Kris, you deserve the best life possible, and you can have that when you help design your own unique and personalized approach to diabetes—when you live life on your own terms. If you have diabetes and are unhappy with your current treatment regimen, overwhelmed by its changes to your lifestyle, or feel guilty if you ever overstep over the boundaries of your care plan, this book is for you. If your diabetes control is fine but you want to enhance your quality of life and feel more positively about your diabetes management, you've come to the right place. If you've ever been told, "No, you can't do that with diabetes," it is time to learn how to say, "Yes, I can!"

I've spent more than twenty years working with people who have diabetes, and I know how frustrating it can be to pursue health goals that don't suit your lifestyle or personality—you may lose the ability to enjoy each day, agonize over test results, fear each medical appointment, get criticized by family members, and feel an overwhelming sense of failure. If you feel this way, you're not alone. According to William H. Polonsky, PhD, CDE, author of *Diabetes Burnout*, about 25 percent of individuals who receive ill-fitting directives ignore them, fail, or quit:

10–24 percent of patients with diabetes reported that they rarely or never followed their health-care team's dietary recommendations.

22 percent of patients reported knowing that they were supposed to follow a certain meal plan, but felt that it was usually or always impossible to do so.

21–25 percent of patients rarely or never followed their doctor's recommendations for blood glucose monitoring.

Sixteen years ago, I developed gestational diabetes and was told to adhere to a strict diabetes regimen—I watched the clock and checked my blood sugar on time, measured my foods, and focused my life around my diabetes needs. I gave birth to a healthy son, but resented the way that diabetes took over my life. After that experience, I pledged to provide my patients with the guidance necessary to help them achieve the quality of life and personal freedom they deserved. I'd like to share this information with you. I'll help you choose goals and diabetes care practices that can work for you. I will introduce you to an array of choices that you may not know about or have never tried. You *can* live a comfortable and fulfilling life with diabetes. To do this, you need reliable information, quality support, and the willingness to work with your health-care team to achieve a common goal—a life with diabetes on your *own* terms. Keep a pen handy as you read through this book. Jot down ideas that you want to implement or discuss with your health-care team. You'll also have an opportunity to "listen" to many diabetes and health experts I've interviewed on my radio show and for the dLife.com Web site. I've included excerpts from these conversations so you can benefit from their wisdom as well. They have much to offer that can help you design your personal approach to your diabetes. Some of the folks you will learn from are:

Betty Brackenridge, MS, RD, CDE, coauthor of *Diabetes Myths, Misconceptions, and Big Fat Lies*

Dr. Stuart Brink, Senior Endocrinologist at the New England Diabetes and Endocrine Center

J. Anthony Brown, a host of *dLifeTV*, and cohost of the *Tom Joyner Morning Show on ABCRadio.com*

Douglas Cairns, the first pilot with type 1 diabetes to fly solo around the world

Fran Carpentier, the senior editor of *Parade*, the national Sunday newspaper magazine

Lorena Drago, MS, RD, CDN, CDE, and author of *Beyond Rice and Beans: the Caribbean Latino Guide to Eating Healthy with Diabetes*

Dr. Steven V. Edelman, endocrinologist and founder of Taking Control of Your Diabetes (TCOYD)

Christine Gorman, senior health writer at *Time* magazine

Dr. Sheldon Gottleib, senior cardiologist at Johns Hopkins Bayview Medical Center in Baltimore, Maryland

Dr. Thomas Hostetter, former director of the National Kidney Disease Education Program

David Kliff, publisher of *The Diabetic Investor*

Mother Love, a host of *dLifeTV*

Laura Menninger, "The Glucose Goddess," a diabetes advocate and comedian

Donna Rice, MBA, BSN, RN, CDE, the president of American Association of Diabetes educators

Daniel Wasserman, DOM, AP, Dipl.Ac., an expert in acupuncture and complimentary medicine

Nina Yarus, yoga and meditation instructor
and many others . . .

This book does not take the place of face-to-face visits with your health-care providers, but it can help you launch discussions that will enhance your diabetes treatment plan.

Remember, this is your life and you should be able to enjoy it as completely as possible. You may have to make some adjustments in order to enjoy certain activities once again, but it can be done and this book will show you how.

Diabetes on Your Own Terms

1

SAY YES TO...
Guilt Free Diabetes Control

ARE YOU READY to love your life again? I'm here to help you do that. Over the years, I've helped countless individuals learn to live with diabetes on their own terms—they travel where they want to go, eat what they love to eat, and feel healthy again. I help them accomplish this goal using three tools: reliable information, enthusiastic support, and Jump-Start Pledges. The Jump-Start Pledge is an easy step-by-step method that I created to help my patients successfully incorporate healthy behaviors into their lives. Follow the same suggestions that I have shared with my patients for more than twenty years and you, too, can have the life you've always hoped for—one with few if any complications and lots of freedom.

IN THIS CHAPTER, YOU WILL:

- Learn how to determine if you are in good diabetes control.
- Discover the value of your A1C test results.
- Choose the best times to check your blood and learn what these test opportunities can teach you.

- Find out different ways to treat abnormal blood glucose levels.
- Learn how to create a Jump-Start Pledge.

STEP 1

Evaluate Your Diabetes Control

>WHEN YOU AIM FOR PERFECTION,
>YOU DISCOVER IT'S A MOVING TARGET.
>—George Fisher

RHONDA *recently posted on dearjanis.com that she has had type 2 diabetes for about six years. She did all that was asked of her and did it well—she went to the gym every Monday, Wednesday, and Friday, and walked with a neighbor on Tuesday and Sunday. She took her medication as directed by her physician, weighed and measured her foods as instructed by her dietitian, read nutrition labels, and avoided foods that could raise her blood sugar level too high. Yet she was aggravated. Her blood sugar level, considered great by most standards, was still not ideal. She expected perfection and felt like a failure every time she tested her blood and saw the result on her glucose meter. It was never where she wanted it to be. In her opinion, things were not going well.*

HERE'S THE FIRST step that will help you improve your life with diabetes. I want you to honestly evaluate how you're doing right now, so you can set personal goals that are achievable. This is a disease that directly responds to your actions. Before you can move ahead, you need to assess where you are and in what areas you desire to improve your health. If you make the right lifestyle choices based upon that evaluation, you will see positive results. On the flip side, if you don't quite understand how diabetes affects your body or how your lifestyle choices may affect you, you may be sabotaging your health despite your best efforts. And that may include trying so hard that you cause yourself unnecessary stress and worry! Don't feel guilty if this happens—remember, we are striving for excellent health, not perfection.

In this book, I will show you how to improve and personalize your involvement with both your health and health-care team, for optimal results. Your ultimate goal is to develop an effective health regimen that you are comfortable with on a day-to-day basis, so you will be able to maintain control over your diabetes rather than letting your diabetes control you.

Is flawless diabetes control possible? I wish it were. But I've never seen it and neither have any of my colleagues. "That's a lot of baloney!" agrees Betty Brackenridge, coauthor of *Diabetes Myths, Misconceptions, and Big Fat Lies*. She feels that none of the tools that we have today can possibly work as well as a healthy pancreas. According to Brackenridge, "Perfect control isn't possible with the tools, even when we're doing everything perfectly . . . and no one does, because we're humans first and we live with diabetes second."

So, how should you evaluate your diabetes control? If you base it on your blood glucose results alone, you are ignoring several large and important pieces of the puzzle. To get a true picture of how you are doing, I recommend you use a great tool developed by the National Diabetes Education Program—the "A-B-C":

A—A1C (blood glucose control)
B—Blood pressure control
C—Cholesterol (and other lipids)

A IS FOR A1C

IN THE WORLD of diabetes, the A1C test reigns supreme. It measures your average blood sugar level for the past two to three months.

Just as the lowly fruit fly has a lifespan of a mere twenty-four hours, the average lifespan of a red blood cell is two to three months. When blood sugar levels run high, hemoglobin in the red blood cells becomes *glycated* (attached to the excess sugar, or glucose). The greater the amount of sugar-bonded hemoglobin, the higher your average blood sugar level.

An A1C test should be taken at the doctor's office every few months. Most experts recommend a target of less than 6.5 to 7 percent. A1C values can be puzzling because they differ greatly from the results displayed on home glucose meters. To better understand your value, compare it with the following chart:

A1C LEVEL (%)	EQUIVALENT TO GLUCOSE RESULT IN MG/DL	EQUIVALENT TO GLUCOSE RESULT IN MMOL/L
6	135	7.5
7	170	9.5
8	205	11.5
9	240	13.5
10	275	15.5
11	310	17.5
12	345	19.5

American Diabetes Association, *Clinical Practice Recommendations 2006*

A result of 7 percent or higher puts you at risk for developing diabetes complications. If your result falls into that category, please explore additional treatment choices with your health-care team as soon as possible.

The A1C is a terrific reference, but it is not perfect. It is possible to have a great result yet not feel well. That is because the A1C represents an average of past glucose results. If your blood sugar level roller-coasters up and down, you may end up with an impressive A1C, yet still have poor control—the frequent highs cancel out the numerous lows. Since this test is only taken once every few months, you must continue to check your blood with your home glucose meter, to keep a close eye on how you are doing. I will go into further detail about the value of your meter later in this chapter but, until then, know that this superb tool puts you in control of your diabetes life. With it, you can make immediate decisions about your diabetes care as problems arise.

B IS FOR BLOOD PRESSURE

UNTIL RECENTLY, IF people maintained a healthy blood glucose level, they probably felt safe from diabetes-related problems. Today, however, we know that good blood pressure control is equally as important as glucose control. Diabetes complications, including those that involve the kidneys, heart, eyes, nerves, and circulation, may worsen if your blood pressure is high. This is because the increased pressure circulates the blood with so much force that it damages blood vessel walls and makes the heart work harder. It also encourages arteries to harden, which can cause cardiovascular-related problems—including heart disease and stroke, the most common causes of diabetes-related death.

What Causes High Blood Pressure?

A variety of factors can cause your blood pressure to climb. These include smoking, obesity, a lack of physical activity, excess salt or alcohol intake, your age, stress, and family history. The most common symptoms include severe headaches, vision changes (which can also occur with abnormal blood sugar levels), chest pain, fatigue, breathing problems, an irregular heartbeat, confusion, and the appearance of blood in your urine. It is also possible to have no symptoms at all, which is why it is so important to have your blood pressure checked at each doctor's visit, or more frequently, if necessary.

Blood pressure is measured by two numbers. The top reading is the *systolic pressure*, which is amount of force that the heart uses to contract and push the blood throughout the body. The bottom number is the *diastolic pressure*, the amount of pressure in the vessels when the heart rests. Take a rubber ball and squeeze it as tightly as you can—that is your systolic pressure. Now release the ball—that represents your diastolic pressure. Most experts suggest that your blood pressure be no higher than 130/80.

The Importance of Keeping It Low

If your blood pressure is in a normal range, that is great. Your risk of developing hypertension will climb, however, if you smoke, have a family history of high blood pressure; are African American and/or older than thirty-five, inactive, or overweight; consume alcohol; frequently eat fatty and salty foods; or are pregnant.

In the late 1990s we learned from the United Kingdom Prospective Diabetes Study that a 10 mm drop in systolic pressure and a 5 mm drop in diastolic helped achieve a 24 percent drop in all diabetes complications and a 32 percent drop in deaths related to diabetes.

Several factors that cause blood pressure to rise are obviously beyond your control. But you *can* do something about many of the causes—and, as this study shows, lowering those numbers even a little may have a huge impact upon your health. In chapters 2 through 4, you will learn how to make some positive changes to prevent diabetes complications.

C IS FOR CHOLESTEROL
(AND OTHER LIPIDS)

FATS OF ALL types, including triglycerides and trans fats, fit into our final category. They are also referred to as lipids. Cholesterol has a bad reputation, but plays an important role in the body—it is used to manufacture vitamin D, hormones, and bile acids, which help digest and absorb fats and fat-soluble vitamins in the small intestine. The two types that deserve your attention are *low-density lipoproteins* (LDL), and *high-density lipoproteins* (HDL).

LDL cholesterol is known as the "bad" cholesterol. Too much of it raises your risk for heart disease. LDL cholesterol is a waxy, sticky substance that travels throughout the bloodstream and adheres to the inside of artery walls, which makes blood circulation difficult. Many experts believe that this build-up happens because a low-grade inflammation is present, from either bacteria or a virus. Clamydia pneumoniae and helicobacter pylori are infectious bacteria that are currently under review; herpes simplex virus and cytomegalovirus are viruses that are also being studied. Depending on what this research discovers, antimicrobial or antiviral treatments may someday be used to help prevent heart attacks. The "good" cholesterol, HDL, carries excess cholesterol to the liver, where it can be removed from the body. It also helps remove some of the cholesterol that lines the artery walls. You must have an adequate amount of HDL cholesterol, or you will have an increased risk of heart disease.

What this means to you, as someone living with diabetes, is that apart from focusing on your blood glucose levels, you also need to pay close attention to your blood pressure and cholesterol levels. This is your best defense against developing diabetes complications that affect your blood vessels and heart.

Triglycerides and Trans Fats

The body stores its extra energy as *triglycerides*. A high level of this type of fat raises your risk for heart disease. *Trans fats* are created when liquid vegetable fats are altered by food manufacturers to become more solid through a process called *hydrogenation*. The words "hydrogenated" or "partly hydrogenated," written next to a type of oil on a product's ingredient list, indicates the presence of trans fats. New nutrition labeling laws require products to include the amount of trans fats that they contain. Trans fats increase LDL cholesterol levels and may also lower HDL levels. Chapters 2 and 6 will explain how you can make sensible changes to your meds and diet, to lower your trans fats and triglycerides

---

**SUGGESTED BLOOD LIPID GOALS
FOR PEOPLE WITH DIABETES**

HDL	Greater than 40 mg/dl (1.1 mmol/L)
LDL	Less than 100 mg/dl (2.6 mmol/L)
Triglycerides	Less than 150 mg/dl (1.7 mmol/L)

American Diabetes Association. Clinical Practice Recommendations 2006

STEP 2
Set Your Personal Blood Glucose Range

NOW THAT YOU have determined your level of control, take the next step and set your personal blood glucose goals. Yes, you *can* help choose your own target range, as long as it fits within the guidelines that have been established by respected diabetes organizations and receives a supportive nod from your health-care team. My patients are initially surprised when I invite them to be part of this decision, but they quickly agree because it makes so much sense. When you are involved in selecting your goals, you are far more motivated to do what it takes to reach them.

The target ranges suggested by most recognized diabetes experts and organizations are generous, and enable you to choose the goals that fit you best, as long as you feel well and achieve an A1C level of less than 6.5 to 7 percent. However, be aware that two major organizations, The American Diabetes Association (ADA) and the American Association of Clinical Endocrinologists (AACE), make recommendations that differ quite a bit from one another as regards blood glucose levels:

THE ADA SUGGESTS:
Before meals: 90–130 mg/dl   (5–7.2 mmol/L)

1–2 hours after starting your meal: less than 180 mg/dl   (10 mmol/L)

A1C: less than 7 percent as a general recommendation, but as close to normal (less than 6 percent) for individuals who can handle it without experiencing significant hypoglycemia.

THE AACE SUGGESTS:
Before meals: below 110 mg/dl   (6.1 mmol/L)

2 hours after starting your meal: less than 140 mg/dl   (7.8 mmol/L)

A1C: less than 6.5 percent

I use both of these recommendations for my patients. The ADA goals are great for those who are newly diagnosed or have difficulty maintaining tighter control. The AACE values work well for highly motivated patients who want the lowest possible risk of complications.

RON, *another visitor to dearjanis.com, has type 2 diabetes. He struggled to control it with diet, exercise, and oral medication. He met with a registered dietitian who helped him create a meal plan, and began to walk for about thirty minutes each day. He noticed a dramatic improvement in his blood glucose level, but his A1C remained higher than he or his doctor wanted it to be.*

They discussed the problem and decided that it was time to try insulin. Tim, his insulin trainer, met with Ron and taught him how to use an insulin pen. He insisted that Ron's postmeal blood glucose level be 110 mg/dl two hours after eating. But Ron couldn't achieve it, despite cutting his carbohydrate portions. He stressed out before every meal. No one wanted to sit with him as he agonized over every bite and worried about the effect that it might have on his postmeal "report card." Each time he drove to the hospital to meet with his trainer, he sat in the parking lot for a while, thinking up excuses for why he had not achieved his goals.

A postmeal goal of 110 mg/dl is an unreasonable goal for most people. It certainly was for Ron. It stressed him terribly and transformed each meal into a personal failure. When I told Ron that he had other options, he was relieved. He didn't know that he could aim for a more lenient target range. I invited him take our first two steps—evaluate his diabetes control, then set his blood glucose goals. Rob set his A1C goal at less than 7 percent and his postmeal goal at 140 mg/dl. He then returned to his insulin trainer and shared this decision; his trainer agreed to the change. With this pressure gone, Rob felt much better, and Tim appreciated his patient's new upbeat attitude toward his diabetes care.

Use either the ADA or the AACE target ranges as your personal guide, or take advantage of the wiggle room that exists between the two. If you start with a higher target range, aim for a lower one when you feel ready. Make the decision that is right for you, and be sure to discuss your goals and how to achieve them with your health-care team.

One word of advice—change may feel strange. When most people move their glucose level into a healthy range, they feel wonderful, energetic, and well. But that isn't the case with everyone:

My doctor told me to get my blood sugar down to about 140, but I can't stand when it goes below 200. When I go lower than that,

I shake, sweat, and get a horrible headache. I'm going to give up and stay high where it's comfortable.
—Louise
(from the dearjanis.com message board)

●

If you feel as Louise does, don't give up—you will eventually adjust to the lower level. Think of what happens to your body when you spend the day in an air-conditioned office, then walk out into the sunshine. Initially, you feel overwhelmed by the temperature change. It may not be that hot outside, but it sure feels that way to you. After a while, you acclimate and feel fine. Don't let unpleasant feelings keep you from making an important change. Just take things a bit slower and allow your body to adjust.

When Should You Test?

There are many moments during the day that make excellent blood-checking times, which we will review in a moment. First, put your results into proper perspective. Your home glucose meter is only a tool to help you make better health decisions—it isn't the school principal waiting to yell at you if you misbehave. Laura Menninger, a diabetes advocate and comedian with type 1 diabetes, believes that her meter plays a unique role in her life:

> In the beginning, I felt really guilty any time I overindulged, and of course, my numbers were higher than I wanted them to be . . . I had to reestablish my relationship and say, you know, it is like a compass to a mountain climber. It just gives you information of where you're at, so you can take corrective action in order to reach your goal. If I were climbing Mount Everest and I was 30 degrees SE of where I needed to be, I wouldn't sit and say—Oh, I stink at this! I give up! I would correct my course and continue on . . . No room for

guilt. That just does more damage. Let's just move on. Do what you can do.

Home glucose meters aren't perfect (they can have a 10 to 15 percent error rate) but provide a great way to identify important trends in your blood glucose control. Use yours often! Here are some suggested testing times that I guarantee will help you improve your diabetes care:

- *Before meals*—This time helps you observe the effectiveness of certain diabetes medications, such as Lantus and metformin, and evaluate how well your body controls your diabetes without the input of food.
- *Two hours after the first bite of your meal*—This time is a favorite of many people. You can see the effect that your food choices have on your blood glucose. Eat a large portion of pasta, and your blood sugar will most likely be higher. Eat a smaller serving, and it should be lower. This test time puts you in control; you can adjust your food choices to achieve better results. It is also an ideal time to see if certain types of diabetes medications are doing their job. Nateglinide (Starlix), repaglinide (Prandin), Byetta, Symlin, Novolog, Apidra, Humalog, and other similar meds help your body handle the carbohydrates in the foods you eat. When working properly, they help you meet your postmeal blood glucose goal. If your glucose level is higher than expected after a meal, do one or more of the following: (a) reduce your carbohydrate food portions; (b) increase your physical activity; or (c) adjust your mealtime medication dose, as directed by your health-care team.

Individuals with type 2 diabetes will often have high postmeal blood glucose levels long before elevated fasting levels appear. Spotting this change can help you begin treatment early.

- *Both before and 2 hours after meals*—Some medications, such as sulfonylureas (glimepiride, glipizide, glyburide, etc.), pioglitazone (Actos), and rosiglitazone (Avandia) improve control during both fasting and mealtimes. If you take one of these medications, test at both a fasting and a postmeal time to monitor its effectiveness. It is especially helpful to test two hours after your meal if you take a sulfonylurea, because it enables you to quickly spot a postmeal blood sugar drop, which can happen with that type of medication. Most doctors will recommend that you test before your meal, but few suggest this 2-hour postmeal test; it is not one that they generally use to make care decisions. I urge my patients to test at this time because it helps them evaluate the impact of their food choices and plan future meals. It can be a great help to you as well.
- *At bedtime*—Everyone should be able to enjoy a problem-free night of sleep. Unfortunately, too many individuals fear that they will wake up during the night with an unexpected low, or sleep through the low and end up in the emergency room. A blood sugar check before bedtime can help you decide what you need to get through the night. If you are lower than your target for that time (for many that is below 110 mg/dl or 6 mmol/L), enjoy a late-night snack. ExtendBar, Nite Bite, Solo bars, and Enterex Diabetic shakes contain slow-release carbohydrates that help maintain normal blood glucose levels all night long. You can also create your own nighttime snack: for every four ounces of reduced carbohydrate yogurt, add one level teaspoon of raw cornstarch. The cornstarch breaks down slowly and helps keep your glucose level within your desired range.
- *In the middle of the night (three AM)*—This time is another great confidence builder for those who worry about

nighttime lows. If your glucose level is fine at three AM, you should be fine the entire night. A check at this time can also help solve a common mystery. If you are all right at three AM but have a higher-than-desired blood sugar level in the early morning, you may be experiencing the "dawn phenomenon." This is a common condition in which the body releases a surge of various hormones during the night that sends blood sugar levels climbing in the morning. A change in medication usually remedies this situation. (To eat a green apple before bedtime has circulated the Web as a treatment for the dawn phenomenon. Unfortunately, it doesn't seem to help. In general, be wary of the Internet variety of old-wives' tales; by trusting in unproven alternative measures, you may neglect using remedies that actually do work or harm yourself.)

- *Before, during, and after physical activity*—Exercise is a powerful blood glucose–lowering tool. Some consider it a form of medication. Most individuals observe a blood sugar drop during and for several hours after physical activity. This happens because exercise improves the body's insulin sensitivity both during and after a workout. Frequent checking helps you anticipate this drop and prepare for it with a handy snack. If, on the other hand, your glucose level climbs after your workout, you may not have an adequate amount of insulin in your system prior to starting your activity.
- *Before driving*—Several years ago, Debbie, a patient of mine, experienced an unexpected blood sugar drop while driving, crashed the car, and was seriously injured. A quick blood check prior to getting behind the wheel could have helped her avoid this accident. Test before getting behind the wheel of a car. If you can't feel your blood

sugar drop, check your blood several times prior to driving. Why several? The blood test that you take only provides information about your blood sugar level at that particular moment; multiple tests will let you know if your glucose level is climbing up or heading down. Some experts suggest that your blood sugar level be at least 100 mg/dl before you get behind the wheel of a car. Speak with your health-care team and choose the level that is right for you.
- If you take care of yourself, you can drive safely with diabetes. Unfortunately, some folks don't realize that. Very shortly, I will share a compelling story of a truck driver who lost his job because of his diabetes. His fight to return to his chosen profession has brought national attention to this issue, and hopefully will educate more people about this topic.

STAY ON TRACK

DO YOU KNOW how to keep your blood glucose level on the right track? I frequently instruct patients who have had diabetes for decades, yet have no idea how to correct abnormal blood sugar levels. They spend years suffering from unexpected highs and lows. Having diabetes without knowing how to treat an abnormal level is like wading in a pool without knowing how to swim. Not only is it dangerous, but it is needlessly restrictive. Once you learn, you can toss away many of your fears, relax, and enjoy yourself more fully. Here are the treatment methods that I teach. They are simple and easy to do. Jot this information down on a card and carry it with you, so you can respond to an abnormal sugar result before it escalates into an emergency:

FOR LOW BLOOD SUGAR LEVELS OF 51–70 MG/DL (2.8–3.8 MMOL/L), USE THE 15/15 RULE:
1. Eat about 15 grams of fast-acting carbohydrate
2. Wait 15 minutes
3. Test again
4. Repeat if needed

Even if your level returns to normal following this treatment, you may be at risk for a repeat episode of hypoglycemia. Follow this snack with an additional one after your next exercise period, during the night, or if you expect to have a delay of more than sixty minutes prior to your next meal.

FOR BLOOD SUGAR LEVELS OF 50 MG/DL OR LESS (2.7 MMOL/L OR LESS), CONSUME 20 TO 30 GRAMS OF CARBOHYDRATE AND FOLLOW STEPS 2 THROUGH 4 ABOVE.

Examples of 15 grams of fast-acting carbohydrates include:
- 3 to 4 glucose tablets (read the package label)
- 3 sugar packets
- 2 tablespoons raisins
- ½ cup orange or apple juice
- ½ cup regular (not diet) soda
- 5 to 6 Life Savers candies
- 1 cup (8 ounces) nonfat milk

When using the 15/15 rule, do not drink or eat more than you need. Stay away from high-fat items, such as chocolate, that slow the glucose-raising effect of the carbohydrate. The uncomfortable feelings that accompany low levels, such as headache, sweating, irritability, and fatigue, take some time to disappear. Your blood sugar level, on the other hand, improves quickly. That is why you should test again after 15 minutes. Once your level is above 70 mg/dl (3.9 mmol/L) or back within your target range, stop snacking. The symptoms may still be there, but if you continue to eat until they disappear entirely, your glucose level will climb too high and the additional calories will cause an undesired weight gain.

There are a few situational variations you need to know about:

FOR HIGH BLOOD SUGAR* PRIOR TO EATING YOUR NEXT MEAL:
- Wait a bit before eating.
- Take a smaller portion of your next meal.
- Do some light activity, such as a brisk walk.
- Break up your upcoming meal into a series of small snacks and save the fruit for later.

FOR HIGH BLOOD SUGAR* FOLLOWING A MEAL:
- Take a gentle walk or do some form of light exercise.
- Drink a generous serving of water.
- Delay your next snack.
- Take additional medication or insulin as directed by your healthcare team, or with the insulin correcting technique listed below.

*High blood sugar is any level above your desired range.

Insulin Correcting

If you use rapid-acting insulin, such as Humalog, Novolog, or Apidra, you can take additional insulin, if needed, to help maintain your blood glucose level within a healthy range. Here is how to determine how much to take:

1. Estimate the number of insulin units that you take in a typical day. Include all types of insulin, rapid-acting and long-acting, in your total.

2. Divide that total into 1,800. (If you use mmol/L as your blood glucose value, use the number 83 in place of 1,800.)
3. Your answer is your insulin correction number—the amount of points that a single unit of rapid-acting insulin should bring your blood sugar down.

WHY 1,800?

The 1,800 rule is an updated version of a guide developed in the early 1990s by Dr. Paul C. Davidson, medical director of the Diabetes Treatment Center at HCA West Paces Ferry Hospital, in Atlanta. He based his original 1,500 rule on observations that he made while working with patients with diabetes. When rapid-acting Humalog and Novolog insulin arrived on the scene, the number 1,500 no longer worked as expected. Through trial and error, 1,800 was chosen as the value to use to determine the sensitivity factor of individuals who use these and other new types of insulin.

HOW ONE PATIENT USES THIS METHOD

Zoe, one of my patients, normally has excellent blood glucose control, but her new job has brought an enormous level of stress into her life. She has trouble sleeping, feels overwhelmed at the office, and is concerned that her new boss may not be pleased with her work. With all that is happening, her blood sugar level has started to run high. Zoe needs to bring it down safely so she can go about her day with confidence. She used to use a sliding scale, but it wasn't precise enough for her. Here is how she now figures out the amount of insulin to take:

- Zoe uses about 60 units of insulin each day.
- 1800 divided by 60 equals 30.
- Her insulin correction number is 30.
- Or, using the alternative method, 83 divided by 60 units

equals 1.4, so if she takes a single unit of insulin, her blood sugar should drop 1.4 mmol/L over a period of 4 hours.

HOW CAN YOU USE THIS METHOD?

A too-high blood sugar count can occur when you are ill, if you've enjoyed too many carbohydrates, if your insulin has gone bad, if your pump is not working properly (or you haven't changed the insulin reservoir in a while), or for no obvious reason at all. Once you determine your insulin correction number, you can correct your blood sugar level in the most precise method that we have right now. Here is the only caveat—this method only works with rapid-acting insulin (such as Novolog, Humalog, or Apidra).

If you use this method, do not "layer" your insulin; that is, inject a dose of insulin while you still have an earlier dose of rapid-acting insulin in your system. Rapid-acting insulin remains active for about four hours. If you take a dose at one PM, but test high at two thirty PM, it may not be helpful for you to take additional insulin—you still have some working in your body. Review the use of your insulin correction number with your health-care team. Don't take more than you need. Keep track of your injection times, and give your insulin the time it needs to do its job.

Periodically review your blood glucose results to search for trends. Do you run higher in the afternoon? Is midmorning a problem for you? These patterns can help you and members of your health-care team make treatment decisions that keep you feeling your best. (If all of your efforts to improve your blood sugar control don't work, it may be time for a different approach, which I'll discuss later.)

CREATE YOUR JUMP-START PLEDGE

YOU HAVE NOW taken the first two steps toward your ultimate goal—diabetes on your *own* terms: you evaluated your diabetes control and chose a blood glucose range that suits your health needs and lifestyle. Now, you need to implement these decisions in a way that works for you. You can accomplish this easily when you use Jump-Start Pledges. A Jump-Start Pledge is a very small and specific health goal that you commit to do for a single week. At the end of the week, evaluate your progress and choose one of the following:

A. Renew your pledge.
B. Change your pledge to fit you better.
C. Add another pledge to your week.

DONNA, *who was referred to me by a colleague, drank five cups of coffee every day. She wanted to quit caffeine, but stopping cold turkey was too difficult, besides which she loved coffee and did not want to eliminate it from her life. So she made a Jump-Start Pledge—to replace one cup of regular coffee each day with a cup of flavorful decaf. She found the change very easy to swallow. At the end of the week, Donna added a second decaf cup to her pledge, thereby reducing her caffeinated intake to only three cups per day. After several weeks of continuing to substitute decaf, Donna was off caffeine entirely, did not miss the caffeine, and no longer had difficulty sleeping at night—all without having to give up drinking her beloved coffee. Jump-Start Pledges helped her successfully meet her goal.*

Too often, we set goals that can't be met. When we fail, we start to lose confidence in our ability to change. An example of this is the New Year's exercise resolution that thousands of people make each year. They purchase new health club memberships and promise to workout regularly for rest of the year. After about a month or two, during which they miss a few workouts because of other factors in their lives, most believe that they have failed, and quit completely. The Jump-Start Pledge starts with a reachable goal, eliminating that sense of failure and building self-confidence. Most people find it easy to keep to a weeklong pledge that fits into their overall lifestyle.

If you can't keep your pledge for a week, then it was probably not right for you—change it and try again. For example:

> TIFFANY, *another patient of mine, pledged to jog thirty minutes every day after work. By the third day, she realized that this wasn't feasible—a thirty-minute jog is more than she can handle. But she hadn't failed—she just needed to alter her Jump-Start Pledge to better suit her physical abilities. Instead of a thirty-minute jog, she created a new pledge—to walk briskly for fifteen minutes after dinner on Sunday, Tuesday, and Thursday. She had no difficulty doing this and felt very positive about her achievement. After seven days, she renewed her pledge for an additional week, and plans to expand the length of her walk to twenty minutes in a few more weeks.*

In each chapter of this book, I'll suggest some Jump-Start Pledges to try. You may come up with some of your own, tailored to your particular activities and needs, after you have thought about what you have read in the chapter. For additional support, please post your progress on the message board at dearjanis.com. I and others will be interested in reading it, and it will serve as a running diary of your own progress.

TAKE CHARGE

CHOOSE HEALTHY GOALS THAT FIT YOUR BODY AND YOUR LIFE.

2

SAY YES TO...
Choosing the Right Medication Options

HERE, WE EXPLORE the medication choices that can help you fulfill your goals.

Before we start, I'd like to share what I tell all my patients: Medications are important, but they can't do their job without your help. In other words, your meds will deliver the ball to you, but it is then up to you to make the right moves to score. You can help your meds do their job by eating right, participating in regular physical activity, maintaining a healthy weight, reducing your stress level, and monitoring your progress. We will discuss ways to accomplish all of these, but first let's meet the meds.

IN THIS CHAPTER, YOU WILL:

- Evaluate if insulin is right for you.
- Follow the adventures of a new insulin pump user.
- Learn about different oral diabetes medications.
- Learn about Symlin and Byetta, herbs, and supplements.

- Explore treatment options for blood pressure and l cho-lesterol (lipids).
- Find out about the "magic pill."
- Choose your first Jump-Start Pledge.

STEP 3
Review Your Medication Options

WHEN *my patient Rayna's type 2 diabetes control became too frustrating, her doctor suggested that she give insulin a try. The idea terrified her. As long as she popped a few pills, she believed that her diabetes wasn't that serious. But to need insulin raised her concept of her condition to a new and frightening level that she could not deal with. She fought off the doctor's suggestion until her control deteriorated so much that she had to give in. The first day was very scary. But with that first injection, she felt an immediate change. She compared it to feeling like a person who has a backache for so long that he forgets what it feels like to be pain-free; her relief came as a revelation. Since that first day, Rayna's improvement has been impressive. Her pre- and postmeal blood glucose levels are within a healthy range, and she has more energy than she's had in a long time. Now she constantly sings the praises of insulin. "I'm so sorry I waited," she says.*

DOES YOUR MEDICAL treatment plan help you achieve the results you desire? If not, it may be time for a change. Diabetes medications range from pills to injected and inhaled products. Don't be shy about sharing a new treatment idea with your health-care team, or about asking them what alternatives may be available beyond what they wish to prescribe. I find it helpful when my patients do that. It shows that they take an active interest in their care and are willing to try something different. Too often, health providers assume that a patient will object to a new or lesser-known approach, so they don't mention it. Don't miss out on an option that might work for you. Yet another way to seize control of your diabetes is to become proactive about whatever substances you take into your body. The following are some choices you may wish to discuss with your health-care team.

TREATMENTS FOR BLOOD SUGAR CONTROL

Insulin

Insulin is a medication option that is available to all individuals with diabetes. If you have type 1 diabetes, you already use it. Your body does not produce this hormone, so you must take it from an outside source to survive. If you have type 2 diabetes, insulin can help you achieve optimal control, especially if other treatments have not succeeded. Sadly, some health-care providers intimidate their type 2 diabetes patients by threatening to prescribe insulin if the patients continue to neglect their health. I believe this tactic is unfair. Insulin is a wonderful product that offers you a chance to feel well again; it is not a punishment nor necessarily an indication that your diabetes has worsened. If you must add insulin to your diabetes plan, you are *not* a failure. It just means that your disease has changed and you require a more effective way to control it.

There are two popular types of insulin: long-acting and rapid-acting. Long-acting insulin, such as insulin glargine (Lantus), is usually taken as a single shot but can be broken up into multiple doses. It helps control the natural blood glucose swings that occur within your body during your waking hours and while you are asleep. But long-acting insulin does not respond to the blood glucose changes that happen when you eat. For those, you need to use a rapid-acting insulin, such as insulin lispro (Humalog), insulin glulisine (Apidra), or insulin aspart (Novolog), which stays active in your body for about four hours. Rapid-acting insulin is usually injected, but it now exists in a new inhalable form that is particularly attractive to people who are needle-shy.

HOW DO YOU FEEL ABOUT USING INSULIN?

To determine how well insulin treatment may fit into your life, select the statement that best expresses how you feel about using it:

A. If I need to use insulin, I want to take as few injections as possible.
B. I will take as many injections as I need to achieve good diabetes control.
C. I don't want to try it at all!

You agree with statement A—If you want to take as few injections as possible, I suggest that you check out the insulin pump. It eliminates the need for routine, daily injections.

You agree with statement B—You don't mind injections, so a long-acting insulin such as Lantus or Levemir, combined with a rapid-acting insulin at meals, can be a winning combination.

You agree with statement C—If you have type 2 diabetes and aren't ready for insulin, that is fine as long as your diabetes care is good. But if your A1C is above 7 percent and you are unable to bring it down with your current regimen, it can offer you enormous help. I encourage you to give it a chance. It takes some getting used to, but you won't be disappointed. Speak with others who have made the transition to insulin. They can help you overcome your fears and concerns. Ask your health-care team to recommend someone to speak with, or visit the bulletin board or chat room at a diabetes-related Web site and ask others posting there about their insulin use.

THE INSULIN PUMP

I love teaching people about the insulin pump. I enjoy the look on my patients' faces when they put the pump on for the first time and correct their blood sugar level with a push of a button instead of an injection. Their euphoria can't be described—suddenly their diabetes is less of a burden. Pump users can skip meals, eat foods that they used to avoid, and sleep without worrying that their blood sugar will drop. The pump is an amazing tool that can be used by individuals with all types of diabetes.

The pump provides insulin in two different ways:

1. It delivers small droplets throughout the day and night, which is known as the basal rate. Its delivery is programmed to the user's exact daytime and nighttime needs. These rhythmic drops maintain blood sugar levels in a healthy range in the same way that long-acting insulin does. The basal rate can be decreased when you exercise or increased if you are ill.
2. It offers insulin on demand. This dose is called a *bolus* and is requested whenever the device wearer consumes a serving of a food that contains carbohydrate.

The pump eliminates the need for routine daily injections, which is a plus for most people. Its infusion set (tubing) and insulin are changed about every three days. The insulin pump is worn day and night and can be disconnected briefly for bathing and sexual activity. It is about the size of a small iPod player and can be worn on a belt, or hidden inside a pocket, bra, or other item of clothing.

THE PUMP IS RIGHT FOR YOU IF . . .
- You are willing to wear a device all day and night (with limited time off) if it helps you achieve excellent diabetes control.
- You want to take as few injections as possible.
- You want the freedom to skip meals and eat a greater variety of foods.
- You are willing to count carbohydrate grams to determine the amount of insulin to take.

- You have frequent blood sugar lows and want a tool that may help limit or eliminate them.

THE PUMP IS NOT FOR YOU IF . . .
- You don't want to wear a device.
- You don't wish to change your treatment plan.
- You don't want to count carbohydrates.

MAKING THE PUMP DECISON

Terry Lee is a regular participant on the dLife.com message board, which I supervise. Let's examine some of the messages that she posted as she struggled with the decision to try an insulin pump, along with some of my personal thoughts about her comments:

> **February 19:** I have an appointment this Thursday Feb 23, to start training for an insulin pump. I am a little nervous getting started on it.
>
>   Thanks for listening.
>
>   TLR

It is natural to be nervous when you begin insulin pump training, so I open my trainings with a few humorous stories. Pumps are made of the same type of material used for motorcycle helmets, so they are almost indestructible. My patients love to hear about pumps that still worked after they fell into cups of coffee, toilets, and yes, even the ocean!

You may wonder how it feels to wear a pump. Most people don't feel it. I wore a pump for a week to learn more about it. I had gestational diabetes years ago, but don't currently have diabetes, so my pump contained a saline (salt) solution instead of insulin. I was pleasantly surprised: I barely felt it at all and had no problem sleeping with it, either—I placed it into a gym sock, pinned it to my pillow, and went off to sleep. There are other ways that you can sleep with it, but that is the one that I tried. A few of my patients worry about what to tell their friends. They don't like the attention that diabetes brings them and don't want to answer questions about any new device. Fortunately, the pump resembles other electronics that most people wear—a cell phone or even a pager. Women who want to hide it while wearing evening wear can even place it into their bra. If you choose to use a pump, you should be able to find a comfortable way to wear it.

> **February 28:** Hi everyone! I get my pump start training on March 14 . . . I am a bit concerned about lows, but I know I will do just fine. I will keep you posted on how I do.

When you use a pump, you must change your diabetes perspective and worry about blood sugar highs rather than lows. With a pump, your blood sugar level will not usually go low. It can if you give yourself too much insulin, but that is a human error. The biggest concern is that your level may go too high. Pumps contain rapid-acting insulin only. If it becomes disconnected or has trouble with its insulin delivery, you will stop receiving insulin. Since you have no long-acting insulin in your system, your blood sugar level will climb.

> **March 3:** I do not know if I will start with saline or insulin. My nurse trainer did not say.

Some people wear their pump with saline solution, in place of insulin, for the first few days. They take their regular insulin injections, but have an opportunity to wear the pump without relying on it for their control. This practice can help you reduce your fears about living with a pump. I don't usually take that step with my patients. I have them start immediately on insulin so they can feel the incredible blood glucose control benefits as soon as possible.

> **March 14:** I'm pumping! I couldn't believe how
> easy it was to insert the infusion set! One try
> and it was inserted.

What stays under your skin when you wear a pump? A flexible, thin plastic straw called a catheter. You do use a needle to initially attach the catheter to your skin, but that needle comes out immediately. Then you connect your insulin-filled pump and you are on your way.

> **March 16:** Last night for supper I miscalculated
> my meal bolus and guess what? When I checked my
> blood glucose two hours after, I was at 62. Low.
> No big deal. I treated with glucose tabs and a
> snack and I was ok.

As mentioned above, human error is what usually causes a blood sugar low to occur. When you wear a pump, you should continue to carry glucose tablets or another form of fast-acting carbohydrate in case of an emergency. You should also be prepared to treat an unexpected high level. If you find that you are higher than your target range, you can use the pump to give yourself a correction dose of insulin. If your blood sugar level is still high when you recheck your blood, it is time to disconnect the pump and take a dose of insulin from a pen or syringe. The pump only gets one chance to bring your numbers back into range. If it is unable to do that, there may be something wrong with the insulin, the tubing, or the pump itself. You will need to carry an insulin pen wherever you go, in case of an emergency.

> **March 17:** I am overcalculating my supper carbs
> and bolusing too much insulin. My trainer said to
> raise my carb-to-insulin ratio. Done.
> We will see how I do tomorrow.

Carbohydrate counting helps you determine exactly how much insulin to take (the bolus) when you eat a food that contains carbohydrate. I describe this method in detail in chapter 3. Most people take one unit of insulin for every 15 grams of carbohydrate that they eat; some use more or a bit less. It takes awhile to learn this technique, but is not difficult to do. Once you master it, it is simple to do, as most people tend to eat the same foods over and over. Once you learn the amount of insulin that you need for these foods, you won't have to redo the calculations every time you eat.

PUMP MODELS

If you decide to try a pump, which model should you choose? All pumps on the market today do their job well and meet strict FDA standards, so you can base your decision on just about anything you wish, including their features, size, colors, and so on. Or just heed the advice of Jason, a dLife.com member, who believes that you should buy the pump "that makes you say, 'Cool!'"

Oral Medication

Numerous oral medications on the market can help improve blood sugar control. They work in several ways:

- Sulfonylureas, such as glipizide (Glucotrol) and glimepiride (Amaryl), help the pancreas release more insulin.
- Meglitinides, such as repaglinide (Prandin) and nateglinide (Starlix), help squeeze additional short-acting insulin out of the pancreas.
- Metformin decreases production of glucose from liver.
- Alpha-glucosidase inhibitors, such as acarbose (Precose) and miglitol (Glyset), block the intestinal breakdown of complex carbohydrates.

- Thiazolidinediones, such as rosiglitazone (Avandia), and pioglitazone (Actos), reverse insulin resistance in muscle and fatty tissue.

If you take a pill that does not improve your control or causes unpleasant side effects, ask to try a different one.

Symlin

Symlin is a hormone that is released by your body from the same cell that produces insulin. It helps to control how your body processes blood sugars, and, because it signals your brain's satiety nerve that you are digesting your glucose correctly, it works as a diet aide. Studies to date have shown that the weight that comes off, stays off.

Dr. Steve Edelman, a noted endocrinologist and founder of the educational organization Taking Control of Your Diabetes (TCOYD), has had first-hand experience with this exciting newcomer on the market:

> I was doing a study on Symlin and my patients kept saying to me, "Gosh, my blood sugars are better, I'm having less highs, less lows, and I'm losing weight." I decided, hey, I want to try it. And since you can't be in your own study, I went to another doctor friend of mine and he let me in as a research participant, and I've been on it for three years . . .
> It's for type 1s and type 2s who are using mealtime insulin . . . If you're a type 2 taking either a premixed twice a day or fast-acting, then that would be a good candidate for you . . . It's an additional injection . . . just like Lantus, it has a different pH than the [other] fast-acting insulins, so you have to take it separately. It means two injections with each meal . . .
> In every single study ever done with this hormone, people have lost weight . . . I lost 14 pounds, and the impressive thing is that I've kept it off.

Byetta

When Dr. John Eng discovered that the saliva of the Gila monster contained a substance that could help those with type 2 diabetes achieve great control, he stumbled onto something remarkable. The Gila monster eats four times per year and stops the release of insulin between feedings. When it eats again, it produces exendin-4 (exenatide), which helps restart the pancreas' production of insulin. Its action is similar to a hormone known as GLP-1, which is underproduced in people with type 2 diabetes.

Byetta is a synthetic version of exenatide. It helps the pancreas release additional insulin, slows down the absorption rate of food, helps you feel full more quickly, and decreases the production of glucose by the liver. Another plus is that Byetta promotes weight loss in most users. If you take Metformin, a sulfonylurea, or a combination of the two, adding Byetta injections to your daily regimen may help you achieve your control goals. Visit cartoonmd.com to view entertaining videos and cartoons that explain how exenatide and other diabetes medications work.

Complementary Options

Herbs and supplements can help you reduce or even eliminate your need for certain medications. Before you try any new herb or supplement—including those that you may wish to take for other medical issues—do the following:

- Tell your health-care team about all of the over-the-counter supplements and herbs that you already use, as many may interact with other medications.
- Use only one new product at a time and watch for side effects.
- Stop taking any new product immediately if any negative reaction occurs, and contact your health-care provider.

- Monitor your blood sugar level more frequently. Treat abnormal levels as instructed by your health-care team.
- Discontinue all supplements several weeks prior to surgery; some can cause complications.
- Check out the safety and effectiveness of products that you wish to try at consumerlab.com or medlineplus.gov.

The following herbs and supplements may help improve your blood glucose control. The typical doses suggested in this list, however, may not be right for you. Discuss the general pros and cons of the product, and the amount that you should try, with your health-care team before taking any of these:

American and Korean Ginseng—May lower blood sugar levels in individuals with type 2 diabetes. Can cause hypoglycemia, nervousness, insomnia, and headaches.
  TYPICAL DOSE: 100–200 mg per day. Many ginseng products contain little or no actual ginseng, so check out reliable brands at consumerlab.com.

Bitter melon—May help individuals with type 1 or type 2 diabetes. High doses can cause intestinal pain or diarrhea.
  TYPICAL DOSE: 500 gm capsule of 2.5 percent extract three times per day, one melon per day, or 2 ounces fresh juice per day

Chromium—Positive effects have been seen in both type 1 and type 2. **Chromium Picolinate is the form that is absorbed best.**
  TYPICAL DOSE: 50–200 micrograms per day

Cinnamon—May help those with type 2 diabetes. Sprinkle a small amount onto such foods as yogurt, cereal, coffee, or tea. Do not use during pregnancy.
  TYPICAL DOSE: About ¼ teaspoon to 1¼ teaspoons per day

Coenzyme Q10—May help individuals with type 2, but can cause diarrhea, nausea, and gastric discomfort. It works best when taken with food.
  TYPICAL DOSE: Between 50–200 mg/day

Fenugreek—Can improve glucose tolerance in people with type 2 diabetes. May cause an upset stomach.
  TYPICAL DOSE: 1 tablespoon of mashed seeds in 1 cup of hot water at least once per day

Gymnema sylvestre—May regenerate insulin-secreting cells in the pancreas. Can lower blood sugar levels in people with type 1 or type 2 diabetes. Monitor blood sugar levels closely, as *Gymnema* may cause a rapid drop to occur.
  TYPICAL DOSE: 1–2 tablespoons fresh leaves, 1–2 teaspoons liquid extract, 2–3 grams dried leaves, or 2–4 g powdered leaves daily

Psyllium—Helps reduce postmeal blood glucose levels in all individuals with diabetes. Do not take along with other medications, as it may delay their absorption.
  TYPICAL DOSE: Use as directed on label

Vanadium—May increase insulin sensitivity in type 1 and type 2, but can cause diarrhea, abdominal cramping, and flatulence. Do not take this supplement if you use blood-thinning medications. Some people have developed a greenish color on their tongue when taking this supplement.
  TYPICAL DOSE: 10–30 micrograms per day

New medications appear on the market almost daily. Many are taken in combination with a different oral medication or with insulin. Ask your health-care team to see if one is right for you.

TREATMENTS FOR HIGH BLOOD PRESSURE

NUMEROUS MEDICINES HELP normalize blood pressure. Beta blockers help the heart beat more slowly and with less force. They also help prevent heart attack and stroke. On the other hand, beta blockers may make it more difficult to feel hypoglycemic symptoms and may make the hypoglycemia last longer.

Calcium channel blockers—Prevent calcium from entering heart and bloodstream, which enables the body's blood vessels to relax.

Diuretics (water pills)—Rid the body of excess water and sodium that cause you to retain fluid and challenge your heart as it circulates blood throughout your body. ACE inhibitors and angiotensin receptor blockers (ARB) prevent the hormone angiotensin from developing and narrowing your blood vessels. The American Diabetes Association currently recommends: "All patients with diabetes and hypertension should be treated with a regimen that includes either an ACE inhibitor or an ARB. If one class is not tolerated, the other should be substituted."

Aspirin—Makes it more difficult for blood to clot, so it can help lower your heart attack or stroke risk. People who have had a heart attack, stroke, mini-stroke, angina, or pain in their calves while walking may benefit from taking aspirin on a regular basis. It is also recommended for individuals who have a history of heart disease, smoke, have high blood pressure, are over forty years old, or have protein in their urine, a sign of kidney problems. If you are taking a blood thinner, however, aspirin may not be for you. Discuss your options with your health-care provider.

Sodium

Should you limit your sodium intake? Probably. Many of us, even those without blood pressure concerns, consume more sodium than we probably should. The 2005 Dietary Guidelines for Americans recommend that our salt intake be limited to about one teaspoon a day, or 2,400 milligrams. If you have high blood pressure, your intake should be limited to 1,500 milligrams, or as ordered by your health-care provider. Scientists at Brigham and Women's Hospital, and at Harvard Medical School asked a group of individuals without diabetes to follow the DASH diet (Dietary Approaches to Stop Hypertension), which is rich in vegetables, fruits, and low-fat dairy products, for thirty days. They found that individuals who switched from a high-sodium diet to a low-sodium intake reduced their blood pressure significantly. Since a reduced-sodium diet helps those without diabetes, you should consider it also. To do this, try the following:

- Use salt-free seasonings in place of table salt. Experiment with natural herbs and spices. See the sidebar on page 37–38 for some suggestions from the *American Dietetic Association Guide to Diabetes Medical Nutrition Therapy and Education*

HERB AND SPICE REPLACEMENTS FOR SALT

For beef recipes try: Aleppo pepper, basil, bay, chile, cilantro, curry, cumin, garlic, marjoram, mustard, oregano, parsley, pepper, rosemary, sage, savory, tarragon, or thyme.

> *For chicken recipes try:* Aleppo pepper, allspice, basil, bay, cinnamon, chile, curry, dill, fennel, garlic, ginger, lemongrass, mustard, paprika, pepper, rosemary, saffron, sage, savory, star anise, sumac, tarragon, or thyme.
>
> *For fish recipes try:* Anise, basil, bay, cayenne, celery seed, chives, curry, dill, fennel, garlic, ginger, lemon peel, marjoram, mustard, oregano, parsley, rosemary, saffron, sage savory, star anise, tarragon, or thyme.
>
> *For vegetables try:* Chili, chives, curry, dill, marjoram, parsley, savory, or thyme.

- Buy low-sodium canned soups, gravies, bouillon mixes, and tomato and vegetable products.
- Limit your intake of prepared and fast-food food items. Many contain excessive amounts of sodium.
- Taste your food *before* salting it. You may need to add less or none at all.

TREATMENTS FOR CHOLESTEROL AND LIPIDS

SEVERAL DRUGS MAY help improve your lipid levels, so discuss your options with your health-care team. These popular treatments include statins, Metformin, fibrates, and nicotinic acid.

Statins—Lower LDL cholesterol levels by inhibiting an enzyme called HMG-CoA reductase, which controls the rate at which cholesterol is produced in the body. They may also reduce triglyceride levels if taken in certain amounts.

Metformin—Prescribed to help improve glucose control, this can also lower triglycerides, LDL cholesterol levels, and raise HDL cholesterol.

Fibrates, such as Gemfibrozil—Help lower triglycerides and may increase HDL cholesterol levels.

Nicotinic acid—Lowers triglycerides and LDL cholesterol, and raises HDL cholesterol levels, but may cause an uncomfortable flushing feeling that can be avoided by taking a small amount of aspirin just prior to the niacin dose. If you have type 2 diabetes, however, nicotinic acid may worsen your glucose control.

Herbs and Supplements

According to the *American Dietetic Association Guide to Diabetes Medical Nutrition Therapy and Education*, the following herbs and supplements may help improve your lipid levels and lower your risk of heart disease. Use them with caution, as mentioned earlier, and be sure to discuss the amount that you should take with your health-care team:

Alpha-lipoic acid (ALA)—May prevent or slow the buildup of cholesterol and fatty plaques on artery walls. This causes hypoglycemia, so monitor your blood glucose levels frequently.
  TYPICAL DOSE: 300 mg per day in divided doses, but doses up to 600 mg daily have been well tolerated

Cinnamon—May improve lipid levels in people with type 2 diabetes. Do not use this during pregnancy.
  TYPICAL DOSE: About ¼ teaspoon to 1¼ teaspoons per day

Evening primrose oil (gamma linolenic acid [GLA])—May help lower triglyceride levels. Discontinue this supplement before having surgery, as it may interfere with healing. It can cause headaches, bloating, and diarrhea.
   TYPICAL DOSE: 360–480 mg per day

Fenugreek—May decrease cholesterol levels, but can cause an upset stomach.
   TYPICAL DOSE: 1 tablespoon of mashed seeds in 1 cup of hot water at least once per day

Garlic—Has a lipid lowering affect, but may cause garlic breath. Do not take with blood thinners and be sure to discontinue taking this prior to surgery, as it may affect healing.
   TYPICAL DOSE: 600–900 mg of garlic powder per day (standardized to 1.3% of allicin content)

Magnesium—May protect the vessels from developing cholesterol and fatty plaque buildup. Can cause diarrhea, nausea, and abdominal cramping in some individuals.
   TYPICAL DOSE: 100–350 mg per day

Psyllium—May lower cholesterol levels in all individuals with diabetes. Do not take along with other medications, as it may delay their absorption.
   TYPICAL DOSE: Use as directed on label.

Fish oils—Can help lower triglyceride levels and may also have anti-inflammatory effect. Discontinue use before surgery. Do not use if you take blood thinners.
   TYPICAL DOSE: 5 grams of combined eicosapentaenoic acid (EPA) and docosahexaenoic acid (DHA) daily. (These are the two types of fish oils that have been studied the most.)

Vitamin C—May help improve coronary artery disease in type 1 and type 2 diabetes. Extremely high doses may elevate blood sugar levels and cause a false diagnosis of type 2 diabetes. Large doses may also cause nausea, abdominal cramps, diarrhea, and gas.

TYPICAL DOSE: 250–2,000 mg per day

Vitamin E—Believed to help reduce risk of coronary artery disease. Do not take large doses if you use blood thinning medications.

TYPICAL DOSE: 200–800 IU per day is considered safe for any person with risk factors for diabetes or heart disease.

THE "MAGIC PILL"

MY PATIENTS ALWAYS ask if there is a magic pill—a once-a-day dose of something that will transform their overall health. Yes, there is. It is exercise. Regular physical activity has numerous health benefits: It improves your blood glucose control; reduces your insulin resistance; tones your heart; strengthens your bones; increases your muscle health and flexibility, and your circulation; allows you to enjoy quality sleep; and helps you feel less stressed and depressed. The euphoric feeling or "runner's high" that people sometimes feel when exercising is usually attributed to the body's release of natural substances called *endorphins*. British researchers recently identified an additional substance that they believe may be the real cause—phenylethylamine (PEA). Related to amphetamines, PEA is a natural stimulant that enters the brain even more rapidly than do endorphins. PEA metabolism is reduced in individuals who are depressed, which explains why exercise acts as an antidepressant. According to researchers at Chicago's Rush University Medical Center, if you offer

PEA to individuals who feel depressed, about 60 percent will show an immediate recovery.

Don't skip your daily dose of your "magic pill." The activity that you do today can:

- Lower your blood sugar levels for up to several days
- Help lower your A1C level
- Increase your insulin sensitivity
- Help control your high blood pressure
- Reduce your risk for coronary artery disease
- Lower your LDL cholesterol and triglycerides
- Reduce stress and mild feelings of depression
- Help you lose weight or maintain a healthy weight
- Improve your quality of life and self-esteem

Find an activity that you will enjoy. If you need prodding to get off the couch, exercise with a partner or join a class. Both can offer added support and help keep you on track. But first review your activity choice with your health-care team to be sure that it is safe for you. Start slow, stretch often, and expand your activity time and intensity.

Several great exercise choices include dancing, tennis, walking, weight training, biking, swimming, water aerobics, tai chi, and yoga.

I'm a big dance enthusiast; I belly dance several times a week. My class times are nonnegotiable—they have the same level of importance as any appointment or work-related meeting. I also try to incorporate physical activity into my social life. Date night for me and my husband begins with a bike ride or brisk walk on the beach. Instead of meeting a friend for lunch, we meet for a walk in the neighborhood.

Try to do at least thirty minutes of exercise on most days of the week, and sixty to ninety minutes if you wish to lose weight. You don't have to complete your workout at one time. If you wish, break up your goal into small, easy-to-handle segments that ultimately add up to your desired total. Slowly build up to your goal. Warm up before you attempt anything strenuous, and remember also to wind down instead of stopping abruptly. Wear appropriate footwear. Physical activity can cause your blood sugar level to drop during and even after your workout, so you may need to adjust your carbohydrate intake or medication dose. If you have type 2 diabetes and control it with diet alone, you aren't likely to experience exercise-related hypoglycemia, but others can use the following guidelines:

- If your preworkout blood glucose level is at or below 100 mg/dl (5.5 mmol/L), consume at least 15 grams of carbohydrate before you begin your activity.
- If your activity lasts longer than 45–60 minutes or is very strenuous, you may need to eat 15 grams of carbohydrate every 30–60 minutes.
- If your activity lasts longer than 90 minutes, take a small carbohydrate snack (about 15 grams) within 30 minutes after you complete your workout. You may also need a snack 2 hours later, as the hypoglycemic affects of exercise can continue for quite a while. Monitor your blood glucose, and treat abnormal levels as needed.

STEP 4

Set Your A-B-C Goals

Now, you are ready to proceed with setting your A-B-C goals. If you can't decide where to begin, I suggest exercise as a first step, because it improves so many areas of the body, including your emotional well-being. Exercise will help relieve much of the panic that you feel about your health, jump-start your weight loss, and immediately improve your blood sugar level.

CHOOSE YOUR JUMP-START PLEDGE

SELECT ONE OF the following Jump-Start Pledge options that follow, or think up one of your own:

- I pledge to walk 15 minutes each day for one entire week.
- I pledge to take my medication, without fail, for one entire week.
- I pledge to check my blood sugar level two hours after lunch [or choose another time] every day for one week.
- I pledge to [your choice] for one week.

Remember, your pledge is for just seven days. At the end of the week, if you feel positive about your new behavior, renew it for another seven days. If your pledge didn't fit well into your life, change it—don't stop setting at least one goal for yourself per week. Once you feel that your pledge has become easy to do, make that goal a little more of a challenge, or add another.

TAKE CHARGE

BE AN INFORMED PARTNER IN YOUR DIABETES CARE. YOUR INVOLVEMENT IN YOUR TREATMENT CHOICES ARE IMPORTANT.

SAY YES TO . . .
Realistic Weight Goals

> I'VE BEEN ON A CONSTANT DIET FOR THE LAST TWO DECADES. I'VE LOST A TOTAL OF 789 POUNDS. BY ALL ACCOUNTS, I SHOULD BE HANGING FROM A CHARM BRACELET.
> —*Erma Bombeck*

THE WORLD HAS defined beauty in different ways over the centuries. When you view paintings by the great Flemish painter Peter Paul Rubens, you see women who looked desirable in his day, but who would be considered a bit hefty by today's standards. Even Marilyn Monroe, who had a voluptuous figure, would be dieting frantically if she were alive right now. On the other hand, today's runway fashion models and magazine cover girls take the definition of beauty to the other extreme: many are dangerously underweight and work diligently to stay that way. Don't evaluate your appearance based on the pages of *Vogue* magazine or the stars of MTV. Look into your mirror and examine your body from a health perspective. Ask yourself a single question—Are you at a *healthy* weight?

IN THIS CHAPTER, YOU WILL:

- Decide if you are at a healthy weight.
- Learn how to use the Body Mass Index (BMI).
- Choose a meal plan that suits you best.
- Find ways to successfully stick with your meal plan.
- Discover how achieve and maintain your weight loss.
- Choose another Jump-Start Pledge.

STEP 5

Set Your Weight Goal

How much should you weigh? How do you know if your current weight is healthy for you? Can you tell by how your clothing fits? If your friends say that you look great, does that mean that your weight is fine? Not always.

When you have diabetes, being overweight negatively affects your health by putting you at a greater risk for numerous medical problems, including heart disease and stroke. If you have type 2 diabetes and your excess weight is stored primarily in your abdominal area, your insulin resistance may also increase, which means that you will require additional insulin to maintain a normal blood sugar level. To get this insulin, your pancreas will start manufacturing even more of it and you may need to take external doses from a pen, pump, or syringe.

Even a modest weight loss of 10 to 15 pounds can help you improve your blood glucose control, normalize your blood pressure, and return your blood fats (LDL cholesterol and triglycerides) to a healthier range. You may also be able to reduce the amount of medication that you take. There are several ways to achieve these goals. However, let's focus first on our initial question—How much should you weigh?

If you employ your bathroom scale to answer this, you'll miss an important piece of the puzzle. Your scale measures weight alone, but that isn't enough; you should also determine if your weight suits your height. For that information, you need to refer to the Body Mass Index (BMI):

COMPUTE YOUR BMI

DO THE FOLLOWING, then interpret your results with the BMI answer guide that follows:

1. Multiply your weight in pounds by the number 705.
2. Divide that answer by your height in inches.
3. Divide that result once again by your height in inches to find your BMI.

BMI GUIDE
   Less than 20: underweight
   20–25: normal
   25–29.9: overweight
   30 or greater: obese

Dave and Gary, two associates of mine, both weigh 185 pounds. That sounds like an appropriate amount to weigh, but as you will see, one of them is overweight. Dave is 5 feet 8 inches (68 inches) tall and Gary is 6 feet 3 inches (75 inches).

DAVE'S BMI	GARY'S BMI
185 pounds × 705 = 130,425	185 pounds × 705 = 130,425
130,425 ÷ 68 inches = 1,918	130,425 ÷ 75 inches = 1,739
1,918 ÷ 68 inches = 28.2	1,739 ÷ 75 inches = 23.2
Dave's BMI is 28.2	Gary's BMI is 23.2

According to the Body Mass Index (BMI) Dave is overweight, whereas Gary is at a healthy weight. If Dave loses some weight, he will reduce his risk of developing health problems.

If you use the metric system, compute your BMI this way:

1. Divide your weight in kilograms by your height in meters.
2. Divide that answer by your height (in meters) once again.
3. Your final answer is your BMI.
4. Use the BMI guide above to see if you are underweight, normal, overweight or obese.

Diane, another colleague, is 1.6 meters tall and weighs 57.1 kg.

57.1 kg ÷ 1.6 meters = 35.7
35.7 ÷ 1.6 meters = 22.3
Diane's BMI is 22.3 (normal range)

If you prefer, you can use a BMI table to find your answer. Locate your height, in inches, in the left-hand column and move across the row until you locate your weight (in pounds). The number at the top of the column is the BMI for that height and weight.

BMI results can be used by most individuals, regardless of whether they have diabetes or not, as a good gauge of whether they need to lose or gain weight. The formula is valid for almost everyone over the age of eighteen, but it does have some shortcomings. It may overestimate the body fat amount of very muscular individuals, such as football players, and underestimate the fat total in older individuals and others who may have lost muscle. If you fit into either of these two categories, discuss your current weight status with your health-care professionals. If you need to lose weight, choose a method that is safe and effective, and which won't harm your diabetes control.

BMI

(kg/m2)	19	20	21	22	23	24	25	26	27	28	29	30	35	40
Height (in.)	**Weight (lb.)**													
58	91	96	100	105	110	115	119	124	129	134	138	143	167	191
59	94	99	104	109	114	119	124	128	133	138	143	148	173	198
60	97	102	107	112	118	123	128	133	138	143	148	153	179	204
61	100	106	111	116	122	127	132	137	143	148	153	158	185	211
62	104	109	115	120	126	131	136	142	147	153	158	164	191	218
63	107	113	118	124	130	135	141	146	152	158	163	169	197	225
64	110	116	122	128	134	140	145	151	157	163	169	174	204	232
65	114	120	126	132	138	144	150	156	162	168	174	180	210	240
66	118	124	130	136	142	148	155	161	167	173	179	186	216	247
67	121	127	134	140	146	153	159	166	172	178	185	191	223	255
68	125	131	138	144	151	158	164	171	177	184	190	197	230	262
69	128	135	142	149	155	162	169	176	182	189	196	203	236	270
70	132	139	146	153	160	167	174	181	188	195	202	207	243	278
71	136	143	150	157	165	172	179	186	193	200	208	215	250	286
72	140	147	154	162	169	177	184	191	199	206	213	221	258	294
73	144	151	159	166	174	182	189	197	204	212	219	227	265	302
74	148	155	163	171	179	186	194	202	210	218	225	233	272	311
75	152	160	168	176	184	192	200	208	216	224	232	240	279	319
76	156	164	172	180	189	197	205	213	221	230	238	246	287	328

SUSAN, *a participant on the dearjanis.com Web site, was quite upset. Her doctor told her that she had type 2 diabetes and needed to lose weight. She had tried many diets over the years, but never succeeded. Now she was determined. The doctor wanted her to see a dietitian and learn how to lose her excess weight at a "snail's pace" of 2 pounds per week. She needed to lose 45 pounds and wanted it off as quickly as possible—2 pounds a week would never do. She drove to the pharmacy, bought several bottles of weight-loss pills and a few packs of meal-replacement drinks, and headed home. She immediately became ill from the weight-loss pills. Her blood glucose level shot up, which made her so ravenous that the meal-replacement drinks did not satisfy her hunger, and she began to overeat. She gained 12 pounds.*

An average loss of 2 pounds per week sounds slow, but is the way to go if you want to achieve a long-term weight-loss success, incorporate healthier eating behaviors into your life, and maintain good diabetes control. Even a weight loss of as little as 10 pounds can help improve your glucose control, lipid levels, and possibly your blood pressure. Slow and steady wins the race.

CHOOSE YOUR PLAN OF ACTION

THERE ARE TWO main approaches to diabetic meal planning, both of which can encourage weight loss or help you maintain your current weight:

A. You change to fit the meal plan.
B. The meal plan is adjusted to fit you.

Plan A

This approach asks you to follow a prescribed way of eating that usually differs greatly from how you eat now. Many diabetes diet books suggest specific eating schedules, food choices, and portion sizes. Some of these regimens are fine, but others may not be safe. Before you start any variety of this diet plan, discuss your choice with your health-care provider. Test your blood sugar often to be sure that your diabetes control is not compromised, and use your common sense. If you don't feel well, your blood glucose level becomes more difficult to control, or you find the program so restrictive that you struggle and cheat, stop immediately.

Avoid any diabetes meal plan that . . .
- *Promises quick and generous weight loss*—Some diets are engineered to kick in an initial high weight loss over the first two weeks, but once the program begins its more balanced phase, the weight loss should slow to a reasonable rate of 2 to 3 pounds per week.
- *Eliminates entire food groups*—Each food group—dairy, grains, meat and meat substitutes (nuts, tofu, and so on), vegetables, and fat—provides important nutrients that your body requires to stay healthy. Limiting is wise, cutting out completely can be dangerous.
- *Makes you feel ill or weak*—A well-balanced meal plan should improve how you feel each day.
- *Compromises your blood glucose control*—This is certainly something that you don't want to have happen.
- *Is too restrictive or repetitive*—You can follow a meal plan that restricts your food choices, but it is very difficult to follow over the long haul. Life is meant to be enjoyed; find a meal plan that enables you to do that.

Choose a diet that . . .
- Uses all of the different food groups, in sensible proportions
- Encourages a gentle weight loss after the initial few weeks
- Feels good while you are on it
- Enables you to maintain a healthy blood glucose level
- Has a comfortable maintenance plan to help you keep the weight off once you have lost it

Plan B

This approach incorporates your food preferences and lifestyle. Enjoy chocolate? It can be included on certain diabetes meal plans. Love pizza? That, too, can be included in the appropriate portions sizes. The "Meal Plan Fits You" approach focuses on your health *and* quality of life. Most people find it impossible to stick to a plan that deviates significantly from their normal routine—they can do it for a while, but soon quit. Plan B works with your tastes and mealtimes to create a diet you can stick to.

Dietitians who are *certified diabetes educators* (CDE) design these types of personalized meal plans. They explore your food preferences, eating schedule, activity level, A1C value, and overall health, then work with you to create a meaningful eating regimen. Once it is established, your insulin and medication needs will be coordinated with this. If you eat on the go, your dietitian will help you choose healthier fast-food options. If you dine out frequently, restaurant foods can be incorporated into your plan as well. If your life includes frequent family dinners and special occasions, you need not forgo them. The ultimate goal is to help you obtain quality diabetes control, meet your weight goals, and have a way of eating that works with your lifestyle.

WHICHEVER MEAL PLANNING approach you choose, remember that the ultimate measure of your efforts is your A1C. As long as you achieve an A1C that is below 6.5 to 7 percent, your choice is probably one that is good for your diabetes control.

STEP 6

Choose the Right Meal-Planning Method for You

THE FOLLOWING ARE several popular meal-planning tools. You can use them to follow a specific meal plan or a personalized plan. They can also be used to maintain your healthy weight, once you achieve it.

THE IDAHO PLATE METHOD

THIS MEAL PLANNING method uses a typical nine-inch dinner plate as a measuring tool. It is great if you are on the go, eat out frequently, or hate to count or measure. It is also quite easy to follow. This plan originated in Sweden and was adapted by members of the Idaho Diabetes Care and Education practice group in 1993.

Here is how you lay out your portions for breakfast:

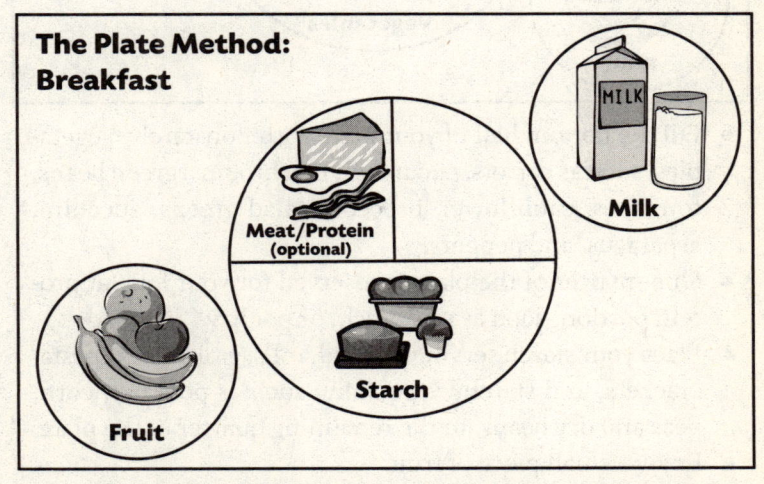

The Plate Method: Breakfast

- Meat/Protein (optional)
- Milk
- Starch
- Fruit

- Use ¼ to ½ of the plate for a serving of bread or cereal.
- Include an 8-ounce glass of skim or 1 percent milk or 1 cup of low fat/low sugar yogurt.

- Add a small piece of fruit, ½ cup of fruit juice, or ¼ cup of dried fruit to the meal.
- One quarter of the plate can be used for an optional serving of meat or protein, such as lean sausage, egg, or cheese.
- If you don't drink milk in the morning, an additional bread/cereal serving can be consumed instead.

Here are the Plate Method portions for lunch and dinner:

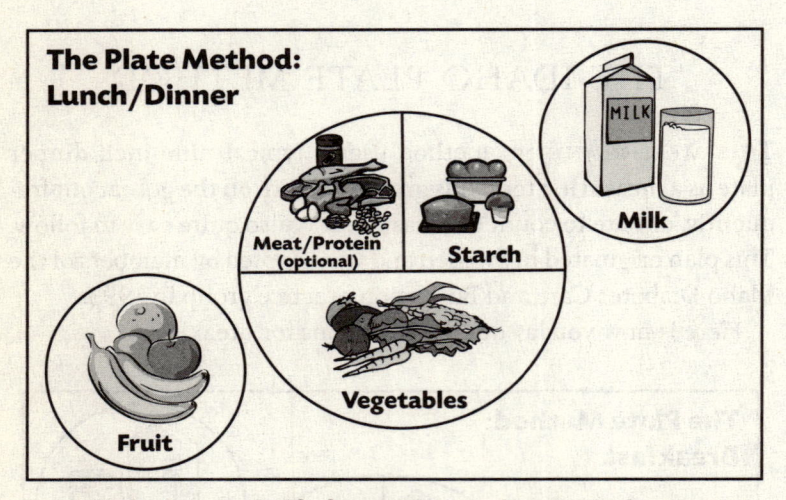

The Plate Method: Lunch/Dinner

- Meat/Protein (optional)
- Starch
- Milk
- Vegetables
- Fruit

- Fill the bottom half of your plate with nonstarchy vegetables, such as carrots, cucumber, mushrooms, green beans, tomatoes, cauliflower, broccoli, salad greens, zucchini, asparagus, and peppers.
- One-quarter of the plate is reserved for your low-fat protein portion, such as meat, fish, or poultry.
- Place your starch serving—bread, rolls, grains, rice, pasta, crackers, and starchy vegetables, such as potatoes, corn, peas and dry beans, in the remaining quarter of the plate.
- Enjoy a small piece of fruit.

- An 8-ounce glass or milk or cup of low fat/low sugar yogurt is included also. As with breakfast, if you choose not to have milk, eat an additional bread/cereal serving in place of it.

A registered dietitian can help you learn this method. For additional meal planning and weight-loss information, visit platemethod.com or portiondoctor.com

THE CARBOHYDRATE-COUNTING METHOD

THIS PLANNING TOOL helps you control your blood glucose level as you achieve your weight goals. If you eat too many carbohydrates, they will raise your blood sugar level and promote weight gain. Eliminating them isn't wise because they are your body's primary source of energy. If you eat about the same amount of carbohydrate at each meal or in a snack, and especially if you tend to eat the same foods frequently, you should be able to predict with some degree of accuracy the affect the foods will have on your blood sugar levels. Sources of carbohydrates include:

- Bread, cereals, pasta, rice, and grains
- Milk and yogurt
- Starchy vegetables, such as potatoes, corn, and peas
- Nonstarchy vegetables (in large servings), such as broccoli, cauliflower, cabbage, lettuce, and tomatoes
- Fruits and fruit juices
- Sugar, cookies, candy, and other sweets

According to the American Diabetes Association, the average woman who desires a weight loss should eat between 130 and 160 grams of carbohydrate each day, and men who want to lose weight should eat between 180 and 210 grams. They caution against diets that restrict total carbohydrate to less than 130 grams per day. Other diabetes specialists may suggest a lower intake. The daily carbohydrate gram amount that you and your health-care team decide is appropriate for you can be spread out throughout the day.

How many carbohydrates are found in certain foods?

The following food items contain approximately 15 grams of carbohydrate when consumed in the serving size shown. (These numbers, courtesy of *Exchange Lists for Meal Planning*, American Dietetic Association)

FOOD	SERVING SIZE
Grains, Breads, Cereals, Pasta	
Bread	1 slice or 1 ounce
Dry cereal	¾ cup
Cooked cereal	½ cup
Cooked pasta	⅓ cup
Cooked rice	⅓ cup
Vegetables	
Corn	½ cup
Peas	½ cup
Potato	½ cup
Other cooked vegetables*	1½ cup
Raw vegetables*	3 cups
Fruits	
Fresh fruit	1 small
Canned fruit (in own juice)	½ cup
Melon or berries	1 cup
Dried fruit	1 cup
Fruit juice	½ cup

FOOD	SERVING SIZE
Milk and Yogurt	
Milk, fat free	1 cup
Yogurt, unsweetened or sugar-free	⅔ cup (6 ounces)
Sweets and Snacks	
Pretzels, chips, crackers	½ cup or ¾ ounce
Cookies	2 small
Ice cream	½ cup
Sugar	1 tablespoon

*Small amounts of nonstarchy vegetables are free

If you eat out or don't have measuring tools handy, use your hand to estimate your food portions:

Your whole thumb = 1 tablespoon
The tip of your thumb (to the first knuckle) = 1 teaspoon
A deck of playing cards or your palm = 3 ounces (the size of a meat, fish, or chicken portion)
Your fist = 1 cup
An open handful = 1 or 2 ounces of snacks such as nuts, cereal, or pretzels.

How to Read the Carbs on Nutrition Labels

Nutrition food labels provide a variety of information that can help you determine your carbohydrate intake. If you are a novice at carb counting, here is how to read the labels:

1. *Locate the serving size listed at the top of the nutrition label*—All of the facts listed below pertain to that serving size. If you eat twice as much, double the values. If you eat half of that amount, cut the values in half.
2. *Locate the total carbohydrate gram amount*—This is the number that you need. Once you find this, you know the amount of carbohydrate that is found in the serving size listed on the label.
3. *Ignore the sugar grams*—They are already included in the total carbohydrate information amount. (Stop here if you need to. Some people find carbohydrate counting a bit overwhelming at first. Once you feel comfortable with first three steps, continue on with the rest.)
4. *Check for sugar alcohols*—If there are any in the product, they will be listed beneath the total carbohydrate value. Add half of this gram amount to your carbohydrate total. Sugar alcohols affect your blood sugar level and should not

be ignored. Their impact is not as great as other carbohydrates, so you only include half of the amount. Examples include sorbitol, mannitol, lactitol, and maltitol. The "ol" at the end of the word usually indicates that the ingredient is a sugar alcohol. These are often found in candies, ice creams, cookies, and other treats.
5. *Deduct some of the fiber*—If a product contains more than 5 grams of fiber, the amount listed can be subtracted from the total carbohydrate amount. Fiber does not raise blood sugar levels. Dietary fiber will be listed beneath the total carbohydrate total.

The Relationship of Carb Counts and Insulin

Carbohydrate counting can be used to determine how much rapid-acting insulin to inject or take via an insulin pump. Individuals who use rapid-acting insulin frequently match their mealtime dose to their carbohydrate intake. Many take 1 unit of insulin for every 15 grams of carbohydrate, but different ratios exist.

If your personal insulin/carbohydrate ratio were 1:10 (one unit for every 10 grams of carbs), how many units of insulin would you take for the following sandwich?

ONE CHEESE SANDWICH	APPROXIMATE CARBOHYDRATE AMOUNT IN GRAMS
Two slices of bread	30
Two slices of low-fat cheese	0
A teaspoon of low-fat mayonnaise	0

If you take one unit of rapid-acting insulin for every 10 grams of carbohydrate (1:10), you would take 3 units of insulin for this sandwich. Now, try calculating the insulin for this meal:

PASTA DINNER	APPROXIMATE CARBOHYDRATE AMOUNT IN GRAMS
1 cup of pasta	45
3 ounces of grilled chicken	0
½ cup of cooked spinach	10
1 teaspoon of trans-fat-free margarine	0
1 small peach	15
1 cup of diet soda	0

The pasta, spinach, and peach are the items that contain carbohydrates. Your total carbohydrate intake for this meal is approximately 70 grams. 70 divided by 10 is 7. You would take 7 units of insulin for this meal.

It takes a bit of practice, but when you match your insulin to your carbohydrate intake, you closely imitate the action of a healthy pancreas, which releases insulin in amounts that the body needs. This method can significantly improve your blood glucose control. It is easiest to count carbs when you use products with nutrition labels, but you can still enjoy homemade products that you whip up in your very own kitchen:

1. Choose your recipe.
2. Jot down the grams of carbohydrate found in each ingredient (use food labels or a carbohydrate gram list).
3. Add up the grams found in each item to determine the recipe's total carbohydrate amount.
4. Divide the total amount by the number of servings that the recipe makes. This gives you your carb gram total per serving.
5. Note that in your cookbook for future reference.

Carbohydrate gram lists are published in many books and can also be found on the Web at www.calorieking.com or www.ediets.com/nt, eDiets.com's free Nutrition Tracker service.

I also recommend that you meet with a registered dietitian who specializes in diabetes, to learn more about how to use carbohydrate counting as a meal-planning tool, and to discuss your diet plan.

If your carbohydrate portions seem limited, you don't have to feel deprived. Lorena Drago, a diabetes educator in New York City, believes that our carbohydrate choices need to change. Lorena believes we should stop choosing starches that are high in carbohydrates, which limit the amount we can take, and select our carbs from a more creative list of foods that offer larger portion options.

Here are a few carbohydrate choices that Lorena recommends:

SERVING	CARBOHYDRATE CONTENT
½ cup spaghetti squash	5 grams
½ cup of pumpkin (fresh, frozen, canned)	6 grams
½ cup jicama (Mexican potato)	11 grams
½ cup chayote	4 grams

Compare these to ½ cup of potatoes, ½ cup of peas, or ½ cup of corn, which each contain 15 grams of carbohydrate. Because they contain fewer carbs, you can increase your portion and place a more appealing amount of food on your plate. Recipes for these foods are plentiful on the Web. Spaghetti squash can be used in place of pasta in many recipes; pumpkin can be seasoned in a variety of ways; jicama can be cut, mixed into a salad, boiled, mashed or baked; and chayote, can be stuffed, boiled, or baked.

Another way to expand your starch portion while maintaining your desired carb total is to add what Lorena calls a "carb stretcher." Mix a nonstarchy vegetable into your favorite starchy one. For example, you can stretch a ½ cup of mashed potatoes into a far larger portion by adding some lightly sautéed portobello mushrooms. Or take that same scoop of potatoes and mix in some rutabaga or turnips. You still eat approximately the same amount of carbohydrate, but now have a more generous amount to enjoy.

THE GLYCEMIC INDEX METHOD

THIS MEAL-PLANNING tool is gaining popularity although it remains controversial. Many organizations worldwide enthusiastically endorse it. The American Diabetes Association has agreed that there is some merit to using it. In their clinical practice recommendations for 2006, they included the following statement: "The use of the glycemic index/glycemic load may provide an additional benefit over that observed when total carbohydrate is considered alone."

The glycemic index (GI) is a list of foods ranked in order of the effect that they have on blood glucose levels. Those with higher GI values cause a greater rise in blood sugar levels, and those with lower values have less of an effect. The right carbohydrate choice can help you feel satisfied, maintain good diabetes control, and lose weight. A precise glycemic effect of a food is difficult to determine, however—its ripeness, cooking method, even the foods consumed with it, can change the value. Because of that area of haziness, some experts question the value of the glycemic index, but many people have benefited from using it, so it appears to have some merit. If you wish to use the glycemic index as a meal planning tool, *The Low GI Diet Revolution* by Dr. Jennie Brand-Miller, Kaye Foster-Powell, and Joanna McMillan-Price, offers week-by-week instructions on how to use the glycemic index to help meet your personal weight goals.

HOW TO STICK TO YOUR MEAL PLAN

ONCE YOU HAVE chosen your plan, it is important to find a way to maintain it with the same enthusiasm as when you first start it. Here are some hints that can help you do that:

- *Enlist a partner*—Find a friend, relative, or co-worker to join you. Update each other on your progress each day. Knowing that you must report to someone helps you stay on track.
- *Post your progress on an Internet message board*—The dearjanis.com message board has a special section in which participants can post their progress or challenges as they try to accomplish their personal health goals. They support each other with advice and personal stories. It is a lot of fun and very encouraging.
- *Keep a personal calendar*—Mark your progress with a star, happy face, or other symbol.
- *Reward yourself for your progress*—Make a list of nonfood prizes: movies, visits to an art fair or tickets to sporting events, a new item of clothing or manicure, a trip, etc. Make a list of possible rewards and earn them.
- *Try an Internet service*—Several online interactive meal planning programs can create a personalized meal plan for you. Many offer diabetes options, recipes, dietitian advice, meal planners, progress tracking tools, and 24-hour phone support. They even offer some flexibility. If you aren't in the mood for chicken on a particular evening, visit your program's Web site and request an alternative choice. Two reliable programs staffed by dietitians who are knowledgeable about diabetes are eDiets.com and southbeachdiet.com.

There is no single diabetes meal plan for everyone. If your dietary regimen is too restrictive, let your health-care team know. Be open about the foods you love and the eating behaviors you enjoy. A well-designed meal plan is comfortable and flexible. A healthy diet is an important part of your diabetes treatment. It can help you maintain blood sugar control and feel your best. And when you feel well, you can enjoy life to its fullest.

HOW TO KEEP YOUR WEIGHT OFF

LOSING WEIGHT IS just the beginning of the challenge. In 1994, Rena Wing, PhD, from Brown Medical School, and James O. Hill, PhD, of the University of Colorado, established the National Weight Control Registry (NWCR), a project that examined successful long-term weight-loss maintenance. The NWCR set out to discover why some people succeed in keeping the weight off, and others don't. The registry has tracked over 5,000 people who are over the age of eighteen and have maintained a weight loss of at least 30 pounds for one year or longer. The average participant lost double that amount and kept it off for more than five years.

The registry uncovered several behaviors that participants use to maintain their hard-earned weight loss:

- They participate in about one hour of exercise daily.
  That is above and beyond their usual activities. Many walk, others ride bikes, and a few run. Several also do light weight training.
- They consume a low-fat diet.
- They eat breakfast every day.
- They are consistent—they rarely deviate from their eating and activity plans.
- Most weigh themselves at least once a week. This helps them catch small weight increases before they get out of hand.

If you have lost at least 30 pounds and have kept it off for over one year, register with the NWCR. Call 1–800–606–NWCR (6927) or visit www.nwcr.ws.

CHOOSE YOUR JUMP-START PLEDGE

HERE ARE SEVERAL Jump-Start Pledges that pertain to this chapter. Hopefully, you have thought of several others that you would also like to try. Remember, only choose one to start with, and keep to it for seven days. At the end of that period, renew it, change it, or add another one.

- I pledge to use the Idaho Plate Method to plan all of my dinners this week.
- I pledge to eat breakfast every day this week.
- I pledge to estimate my carbohydrate intake for every lunch that I eat this week.
- I pledge to [your choice] for one week.

TAKE CHARGE

DESIGN A DIET THAT WILL MAINTAIN A HEALTHY BLOOD GLUCOSE LEVEL AND HELP YOU MAINTAIN A HEALTHY WEIGHT FOR YEARS TO COME.

4

SAY YES TO...
A Life with Few or No Diabetes Complications

I am twenty-three years old and have had type 1 diabetes for ten years, but I ignore it most of the time. I just don't want to deal with it. My endocrinologist was constantly on my back to take better care of myself, but I never listened to his warnings. Now I am afraid that I'm getting some horrible health problems and just don't want to think about it.
—Jane

ARE YOU AFRAID of developing diabetic complications? My patients certainly are, and with good reason. Each one of them can tell you stories about a loved one or acquaintance who suffered through an amputation, became blind, or died at a young age. They fear that the same will happen to them. Fortunately, diabetes care has changed dramatically in the past few years. We know more about diabetes than ever before, and can say with confidence that *diabetes complications are not inevitable*.

We've already discussed some tools that you can employ to prevent or delay diabetes complications, including regular physical activity, weight control, meal planning, and medications. Now, let's examine these complications. The more you know about them, the more motivated you will become toward reaching your healthcare goals. As we go along, I'll share additional treatments that you may not be aware of and suggest several Jump-Start Pledges to add to your list.

IN THIS CHAPTER, YOU WILL:

- Learn about long-term complications of diabetes.
- Discover what you can do to help avoid or delay these complications.
- Choose another Jump-Start Pledge.

STEP 7

Learn about Possible Complications and

STEP 8

Choose Treatments that Will Work for You

COMPLICATIONS FROM DIABETES include diseases of the heart and blood vessels, eyes, kidneys, nerves, feet, skin, and gums. The exact cause of many of these problems is not yet known, but what is known is that it is not healthy to have excess glucose in your bloodstream for an extended period of time. It interferes with the ability of certain cells to work properly, can cause cells to swell and become damaged, and promotes the production of advanced glycated end products (AGEs) that injure cells and tissues. If you maintain good blood glucose control, keep your blood pressure in an optimal range, stay physically active, achieve a healthy weight, make beneficial food choices, and don't smoke, you significantly reduce your risk for developing complications. Let's examine some of these diabetes-related problems, and the actions that you can take to prevent or delay them.

YOUR HEART AND BLOOD VESSELS

PEOPLE WITH DIABETES have a greater risk of developing coronary artery disease, a progressive narrowing of the arteries, which occurs when LDL cholesterol and triglycerides deposit on the inside of blood vessel walls. Think of your garden hose. If dirt cakes on the inside, it will impede the flow of water—clear it out and the water will flow smoothly. Deposits inside of the blood vessels can slow down or even stop blood from circulating throughout the body. If the heart doesn't receive enough blood, a heart attack can happen. If blood flow is reduced to the brain, a stroke may occur. Decreased blood flow to your feet and legs will prevent wounds from healing quickly, and inadequate blood flow to the penis will make it more difficult for a man to achieve or maintain an erection.

Some researchers believe that LDL cholesterol poses a double threat: it not only narrows the insides of blood vessels but may also tear nearby tissue as it expands and solidifies. Obesity, high blood pressure, a low level of HDL cholesterol (which removes bad cholesterol), lack of physical activity, and smoking, all increase the risk of developing heart disease.

Smoking in particular raises blood pressure, reduces the flow of blood in the arteries, increases the likelihood of developing blood clots, heightens the potential need for amputations, and can increase the risk of erectile dysfunction (ED) in men. If you smoke, stop. It will significantly improve your health and reduce your risk of developing many long-term complications of diabetes. Dr. Sheldon Gottlieb, senior cardiologist at Johns Hopkins Bayview Medical Center in Baltimore, Maryland, shares his thoughts on this habit:

Smoking is a major problem. There's really not much that you can say in favor of smoking. . . . It makes the arteries worse, it makes the good cholesterol lower, it worsens blood sugar control, it smells, and quite frankly is very disgusting and also is very expensive. We usually see, in our coronary care unit, people who have smoked a half a million to three quarters of a million cigarettes during their lifetime. That is a huge number of cigarettes.

Smoking impacts on all areas of your health. There are numerous approaches that can help you stop this habit, including patches, pills, gums, even hypnosis and acupuncture. Discuss these choices with your health-care team and choose a plan that will work for you.

Heart-Healthy Solutions

ENJOY TWO MEALS OF FISH EACH WEEK

Certain fish contain large amounts of two types of omega-3 fatty acids, eicosapentaenoic acid (EPA) and docosahexaenoic acid (DHA), which help block dangerous irregular heart rhythms and prevent sudden cardiac death. These fish include:

- Salmon
- Mackerel
- Lake trout
- Herring
- Sardines
- Albacore tuna

If you dislike fish or wish to take a more concentrated dose of fish's beneficial omega-3 fatty acids or flavored fish oil capsules are a good choice. Some studies show that an intake of 3 grams of fish oil per day can reduce triglyceride levels by 30 percent. Omega-3 may interfere with aspirin and clotting medications. [If you cur]rently take any of these drugs, review your use of fish [oil with your] health-care team. Also, not all fish oils on the mark[et are proven] safe. Search for a brand that bears the Consumerlab.com seal of approval or is endorsed on its Web site, www.consumerlab.com. They test popular supplements for safety and effectiveness.

LIMIT YOUR INTAKE OF CHOLESTEROL AND OTHER UNHEALTHY FATS

One way to reduce your cholesterol level is to reduce (not eliminate) your intake of cholesterol-containing foods, such as

- Animal fats
- Butter
- Cream
- Fat in dairy products

Low-fat and fat-free versions of these foods have little if any cholesterol and are fine to eat. Although egg yolks contain cholesterol, they raise both HDL and LDL cholesterol levels, so many experts have relaxed their restriction and permit whole eggs on diabetic meal plans.

Cholesterol-rich foods also contain saturated fat, which, along with trans-fatty acids or "trans fats," significantly increase the body's blood cholesterol level and should be limited or avoided. Saturated fats are also found in coconut oil, palm oil, palm kernel oil, and cocoa butter. Trans fats are created when hydrogen is added to vegetable oils to make them more useful in commercial food preparation. Cookies, French fries, crackers, doughnuts, and other similar products often contain trans fats. Nutrition food labels list the presence of trans fats in a product, so inspect grocery items as you shop and choose wisely.

The American Heart Association, the American Diabetes Association, and National Cholesterol Education Programs all have similar recommendations for fat intake:

Saturated fat intake—less than 10 percent of your total calories per day

Cholesterol intake—less than 300 mg per day

If your LDL cholesterol is 100 mg/dl or higher, you should reduce your saturated fat intake to less than 7 percent of your total daily calories and reduce your dietary cholesterol intake to less than 200 mg per day. Visit the comprehensive National Cholesterol Education Program's Therapeutic Lifestyle Changes Web pages at www.nhlbi.nih.gov/chd/lifestyles.htm. This interactive program can help you plan your food choices and help you reach your personal cholesterol lowering goals.

USE HEALTHIER FATS AND OILS

Dress your salad (and other foods) with healthy oils. For all of your cooking needs, choose those that contain 2 grams or less saturated fat per tablespoon. Canola, grape seed, and olive oils are great choices. Sesame oil may help lower high blood pressure and reduce the amount of hypertension medication that you need.

Increase your intake of monounsaturated fatty acids. They help reduce LDL cholesterol levels without lowering your important HDL level. Foods that are rich in monounsaturated fatty acids include olive, peanut, and canola oil; cashews, peanuts, pistachios, olives, and avocados.

Polyunsaturated fats can be included in your diet, but they lower both LDL and HDL cholesterol levels. They are found in safflower, sunflower, corn, and soybean oils; margarines that are created from these oils; Brazil nuts, walnuts, and most brands of mayonnaise.

EAT GARLIC AND HOT PEPPERS

Garlic contains a substance called *allicin* that encourages a short-term decrease in total cholesterol and triglycerides levels. Throw some garlic into different foods that you eat. Add some to your soups, sauces, salad dressings, stews, vegetable dishes, gravies and sauces, and more. If you aren't a fan of garlic, try roasting some:

> Every weekend I roast several heads of garlic, and then keep them refrigerated and add them to soups, sauces, etc.—the roasting mellows the edge that most fresh garlic has, as well as the pungent smell/taste (which I don't really mind—but because I do eat a lot of garlic, I've come to prefer roasted to fresh). It takes very little (active) time, only about an hour in the oven, and keeps in the fridge for at least a week, in a covered container.
> —Matthew

If you prefer to take garlic supplements, search for a brand that has the Consumerlab.com approval. Discontinue taking garlic a few weeks prior to having any surgical procedure, as it can thin the blood and make healing more difficult.

ALTER YOUR CARB CHOICES

When you keep your carbohydrate intake at a healthy level and choose more whole-grain versions of your favorite carbohydrate foods, you can help improve your blood glucose control, lower your risk for diabetes-related complications, and feel more satisfied. According to a study conducted at Johns Hopkins University, a meal plan in which carbohydrate foods are partially replaced with protein or monounsaturated oils (such as olive and canola), whole rather than processed grains, and various nuts and seeds can improve your blood pressure, lipid level (fats in the bloodstream), and lower your risk for heart-related problems.

A moderate carbohydrate intake can also help you meet your weight goals. Diabetes meal approaches run the gamut from extremely low carbohydrate to generously high. There may be merit in putting the brakes on an overly generous carbohydrate intake, but don't eliminate carbohydrates altogether—they supply the type of energy that your brain and the rest of your body prefer to use.

Healthy carb-containing choices include:

- Brown rice
- Whole-grain pasta
- Whole-grain cereal
- Fruit
- Vegetables
- Low-fat milk and yogurt

LIMIT YOUR "CUP O' JOE" AND WINE

Coffee is an enigma. Some studies associate it with an increase in heart disease, whereas others say that it is not harmful at all. A recent Swiss study ruled out caffeine as the ingredient that causes cardiovascular problems; the harmful ingredient, however, remains unknown, and may be in both decaf and regular coffee. Decaffeinated coffee can increase LDL cholesterol levels, and the caffeine in regular coffee may raise blood glucose levels. What should you do? If you drink one or two cups of decaf or regular coffee each day, you probably have nothing to worry about. If your intake is greater than two cups per day, it might be wise to cut back.

YOUR EYES

IF YOUR EYES are exposed to high levels of glucose over a period of years, two significant problems can develop:

- Background retinopathy
- Proliferative retinopathy

In background retinopathy, small blood vessels in the retina weaken, balloon out, and burst, leaking fluid and blood into the area. If this happens, your vision can be affected.

In proliferative retinopathy, the eye grows additional blood vessels when damaged ones are unable to bring enough oxygen to the tissues of the retina. These new vessels are fragile and may leak as well. If left untreated, they will continue to bleed and create scar tissue. As the scar tissue contracts, it can tear the retina and cause it to separate from the back of the eye, causing blindness. Other common eye problems include cataracts and glaucoma. You may also experience occasional blurring if your blood sugar level runs high, but that is a temporary situation that remedies itself once your level returns to normal. If you are concerned, speak with your doctor.

Eye-Healthy Solutions

There are no retinopathy medications, so have your eyes checked regularly. This way, any problems can be dealt with immediately. If discovered early, leaking blood vessels can usually be sealed up with a laser. More complex problems may require surgery. If you have type 1 diabetes, visit a qualified ophthalmologist or optometrist within three to five years of your initial diagnosis of diabetes for a dilated eye exam. If you have type 2, get a dilated exam as soon as possible after your diagnosis. Once you have that initial exam, see your eye care specialist annually, regardless of the type of diabetes that you have. Maintain a healthy blood pressure, don't smoke, and if you do develop retinopathy or cataracts, speak to your health-care professional about *bilberry*, an herb that may help improve your condition.

YOUR KIDNEYS

KIDNEYS FILTER BLOOD. They keep the important substances like protein in, and send the waste products out of the body as urine. With diabetes, the small blood vessels in the kidney can thicken, which prevents them from filtering properly. Diabetes-related kidney disease is called *nephropathy*. The earliest sign of nephropathy is the appearance of a small amount of protein in your urine. There are no symptoms or changes that you will see or feel on your own, so regular testing is critical. Each year, your physician should measure the amount of protein in your urine and evaluate the health of your kidneys.

Dr. Thomas Hostetter, the former director of the National Kidney Disease Education Program, offers these additional comments:

> [When] the kidney's filtration is low or there's excess albumin in the urine, it's a signal to think again about how good your glycemic control is, because we know that even ratcheting up glycemic control after there's kidney damage can prevent or slow damage. And second, we know that once those evidences of kidney damage are there, really good control of blood pressure is important.

Kidney-Healthy Solutions

You may have heard that you can protect your kidneys if you reduce your protein intake. There is some evidence that supports that practice, but most of it isn't as compelling as the studies that show the protective effects that improved blood pressure and blood sugar have on kidney health. Most experts recommend a protein intake of 1 gram a day per kilogram body weight. That amounts to about 60 to 70 grams per day for the average adult. Many experts believe that high-sodium diets promote high blood pressure, so ask your health-care team if you should limit your salt intake. (See chapter 2 for additional ways to improve your blood pressure.)

YOUR NERVES

DIABETES CAN ALSO affect the nerves throughout your body. Diabetic nerve disease, known as *neuropathy*, damages the peripheral nerves in the legs, feet, and hands, as well as the *autonomic nerves* that regulate different actions inside of your body, such as the digestive system, heart, bladder, bowel, ability to sweat, and sexual response.

SYMPTOMS OF PERIPHERAL NEUROPATHY INCLUDE:
- Numbness
- Pain
- Tingling
- Decreased sensation
- Muscle weakness

AUTONOMIC SYMPTOMS INCLUDE:
- Nausea
- Vomiting
- Stomach distension
- Constipation
- Diarrhea
- Incontinence
- Dizziness

Sexual problems can occur as well. Fifty percent of men with diabetes have difficulty maintaining an erection. For some, this develops because their nerves are damaged and can't deliver sexual messages properly. Thirty percent of women with diabetes have trouble becoming aroused during sexual activity—they may lack adequate vaginal lubrication and have difficulty achieving orgasm. These issues can be exacerbated by nerve damage. Unfortunately, these issues are rarely discussed during physician visits that are taken up with dealing with such issues as your blood glucose level, blood pressure, or circulatory system. And, as sexual performance is such a personal issue, you may feel uncomfortable admitting to your regular physician that you are having problems in this area of your life—doubly so if the doctor's first try at solving your difficulty hasn't helped. As Donna Rice, an expert in the area of diabetes and men's sexual health, explains, "Oftentimes, men will go to the physician and may get a [prescription] for Viagra or Cialis or Levitra . . . but if it doesn't work, there's no conversation or follow-up as to the effects of that."

Many excellent treatments for the sexual complications of diabetes are available, so don't be shy. Discuss them with a member of your health-care team, or ask for a referral to someone who specializes in this area. Treatments may include pills, injections, penile suppositories, vacuum pumps, lubricants, and counseling, which are discussed in greater detail in chapter 7. If one doesn't work for you, try another. You will find something that may not give you the exact performance level that you hoped for, but you will be able to resume an enjoyable intimate life.

Nerve-Healthy Solutions

To help relieve the tingling, burning, and pain of neuropathy, you may find the following supplements and treatments helpful in addition to prescription medications that your physician may suggest:

- Alpha-lipoic acid supplements
- Evening primrose oil capsules
- Capsaicin (cayenne pepper) topical cream; this may take several weeks to take effect
- Hypnosis
- Biofeedback training
- Acupressure
- Acupuncture
- Anodyne therapy—an infrared light treatment

ACUPUNCTURE

An ancient treatment used in Chinese medicine, acupuncture is now accepted by most medical professionals as an effective therapy for pain. During a treatment session, sterile, thin metal needles are inserted into different areas of the body along special pathways called *meridians*. In Chinese medicine, the body's healing energy or "Qi" (pronounced "chee") flow through these pathways. Acupuncture needles help promote the proper flow of Qi, lower blood glucose levels, and significantly reduce the discomfort of diabetic neuropathy in many individuals.

Daniel Wasserman is a respected acupuncture therapist and Chinese medicine practitioner in south Florida. He treats individuals for a variety of different medical conditions. He believes that this ancient treatment offers a meaningful option to all individuals:

> Most things can heal, but sometimes the body needs a little "nudge." Acupuncture provides that "nudge." It stimulates the body at key strategic points to stimulate blood flow, nerve flow, lymph, in order for the body to heal itself . . . Right now, it's the most referred to alternative medicine in America. There's been tons of research now, not so much asking, "Does it work?"—that's pretty much now accepted—but how it works . . . Locally, it stimulates blood flow to areas that don't get a lot

of that like cartilage, ligaments, bones. At the same time, it's a great physical therapy tool to relax muscles. We know systemically, it stimulates things like endorphins that help with pain . . . it helps nerve regeneration. It seems to work on multiple levels . . . I've always worked with other conventional medical doctors, because there's only one type of medicine out there—whatever is in the best interest of that patient.

YOUR FEET

DIABETIC FEET REQUIRE special attention. They can lose sensitivity, have circulation problems, experience a reduced ability to fight infections, and develop ulcers that may lead to amputations. Good care can help reduce or prevent many of these issues.

> TANYA *was on the way to the mall, when she stepped on a tack that pierced the bottom of her sandal and entered her foot. She didn't feel a thing. She has type 2 diabetes and knows that it is possible to lose sensitivity in her feet, but because she has never experienced any numbness, she never checks her feet or gives them any special attention. Ideally, we should feel pain when we are injured. Tanya did not feel any, so she continued shopping. When she arrived home, she spotted some blood on the bottom of her foot, found the cut, and immediately attended to it. If she hadn't noticed the blood, she could have ignored her foot altogether and the injury could have grown into a sizeable infection and caused incredible damage.*

Ulcers form on your feet when they are subjected to a constant amount of or a sudden increase in pressure. This can happen if your shoes become too tight or begin to rub in a particular spot. If ignored or missed, an ulcer, just like an untreated cut, can become infected, spread, and damage your limb so dramatically that you face a possible amputation.

Feet-Healthy Solutions

Do the following to keep your feet safe:

- *Check your feet each day*—Examine the top, bottom, and between the toes, for redness, cuts, blisters, cracks, and other injuries, and treat them as directed by your health-care team. If you have difficulty inspecting your feet, use a mirror or enlist the help of a friend.
- *Choose comfortable shoes*—Don't buy a stiff, uncomfortable pair and expect to break them in. They should feel good when you first put them on. Athletic shoes and soft leather ones are good for daily wear.
- *Get used to new shoes slowly*—Wear them for a brief amount of time around the house (about one hour) for several days in a row. Check for any redness or discomfort. Gradually increase your wearing time.
- *Shake out your shoes before wearing them*—You may not notice a pebble or small item that has fallen inside.
- *Wash your feet daily*—Use a gentle soap and dry them carefully, especially between the toes. Moisture encourages the growth of bacteria that may cause infection.
- *Moisturize*—Keep your feet supple. Use a moisturizer prepared especially for diabetic skin. Do not use it between your toes unless the package states that you can do so. Moisture should be avoided in that area, as mentioned above.
- *Don't attempt any home surgical procedures*—Don't shave down calluses, clip ingrown toenails, or try to trim excess skin. Have your podiatrist take care of these issues, and inform him or her that you have diabetes, so that your feet will be given particularly careful treatment.
- *Always wear footwear, even while at home*—There is always a risk that you may step on a sharp object and develop an infection.
- *Have your doctor check your feet at each visit*—Remove your

shoes and socks when you enter the exam room. That will remind your doctor to inspect them.

YOUR SKIN

A VARIETY OF different skin problems may occur when you have diabetes. Several can be avoided or improve with good diabetes control. Here are a few of the most common:

- *Acanthosis nigricans*—This is a dark pigmentation on the back of the neck and under the arms. It is usually a sign of insulin resistance and is commonly seen in children with type 2 diabetes. There is no treatment.
- *Alopecia (hair loss)*—This is sometimes seen in individuals with type 1 diabetes. The cause is not known.
- *Dry skin*—Diabetic nerve damage makes it more difficult for your body to sweat. It can also occur if your blood sugar level is high and you urinate frequently. Dehydration can cause your skin to become dry. Use a moisturizer, maintain a healthy blood sugar level, and be sure to drink an adequate amount of fluids.
- *Fungal infections*—Diabetes puts you at a greater risk of developing fungal problems, especially between your toes and in the creases of your body. Maintain your blood sugar level in a healthy range to reduce your risk.
- *Necrobiosis lipoidica diabeticorum* (also known as simply *necrobiosis*)—This is a skin condition that affects the shins and lower legs, that is related to a change in the collagen under the skin. The skin becomes thick and reddish-brown, and may develop ulcers. It is seen more frequently in women than men. Steroid injections may help.
- *Pruritus (itchy skin)*—This can have several causes including

nerve damage, kidney problems, and shingles, which are common in people with diabetes. Seek an accurate diagnosis. If you are developing kidney problems, they must be treated as soon as possible.
- *Thick skin*—People who have had diabetes for more than 10 years, may experience a thickening of their skin. The cause is not known.
- *Xanthelasmas*—These are small yellow plaques that appear on the eyelids and are caused by high blood glucose and lipid levels. They may improve when your glucose, cholesterol, and triglyceride levels return to a healthy range.
- *Vitiligo (a loss of skin pigment)*—This develops in individuals with type 1 diabetes. It appears to go hand-in-hand with the autoimmune nature of the disease. It cannot be prevented.

Skin-Healthy Solutions

Along with the specific treatments detailed above, controlling your blood sugar, blood pressure, and lipid levels will help you avoid skin problems. Drink an adequate amount of water, especially when you exercise or engage in other strenuous activity. Keep your body's folds and crevices clean and dry, to prevent the development of fungal infections.

YOUR GUMS

IF YOUR DIABETES is not well controlled, problems can develop in your mouth, including sores that won't heal, bleeding gums, bad breath, infections, gum disease, and cavities. Diabetes-related nerve damage can cause you to feel a numb or burning sensation in your mouth, and reduce your saliva production. This increases your risk of developing a dry mouth, oral infections, and cavities. Elevated blood sugar levels can also affect circulation and healing, and increase your chance of developing various oral fungal infections, such as thrush. If left untreated, thrush, whose symptoms include red irritated skin or creamy white patches in the mouth, can cause your blood sugar levels to swing.

Mouth-Healthy Solutions

Have your teeth cleaned and checked at least every three to six months, or as often as directed by your dentist. If you have any problems, such as bleeding gums, bad breath, or dry mouth, make an appointment as soon as possible. When you are ready for your visit, do the following:

- *Tell your dentist you have diabetes*—He or she may choose a shorter-acting anesthetic, so you won't have to postpone your next meal.
- *Eat before your appointment*—The best time to have dental work done is when your blood sugar level is in a normal range. If you take insulin, a morning visit after breakfast is a great time.
- *Try to stay on your regular meal plan following dental work*—If you are unable to chew for a period of time, eat softer or liquid foods. Liquid meal-replacement drinks designed for diabetics are a good choice.
- *Delay dental surgery until your blood sugar is under control.*
- *Brush your teeth at least twice a day and floss daily*—Use a soft-bristled toothbrush and replace it when the bristles wear out.
- *Do not use any mouthwash that contains alcohol*—Alcohol may irritate your mouth. If you have a persistent case of bad breath, normalize your blood sugar levels and contact your dentist for assistance.

- *Prevent dry mouth*—If your mouth is dry, sugarless gums and candies will help stimulate the flow of saliva and reduce the formation of cavities. Water and ice can temporarily be used to moisten your mouth. Your dentist can also provide you with special gels and rinses that should help.

DIABETIC COMPLICATIONS DON'T have to become part of your life. If you have already developed some complications, there are many things you can do to help slow their progress. If you haven't experienced any complications, stay on top of your health to prevent or stall their occurrence.

CHOOSE YOUR JUMP-START PLEDGE

- I pledge to check my feet before bedtime for one week.
- I pledge to wear footwear all day for one week.
- I pledge to floss my teeth once a day for one week.
- I pledge to switch to low-fat dairy products for one week.
- I pledge to eat fish twice this week.
- I pledge to start a smoking cessation program this week.
- I pledge to [your choice] for one week.

TAKE CHARGE

MANY DIABETES COMPLICATIONS CAN BE PREVENTED OR HALTED BY TAKING GOOD CARE OF YOUR BODY.

5

SAY YES TO . . .
Getting the Guidance You Need

WHEN KAREN, A patient of mine, spotted an enticing weight-loss advertisement in a respected diabetes magazine, she asked me for my opinion. I've been a member of the American Diabetes Association advertising review panel for several years and am pretty tough when it comes to ad approval. This one didn't meet my standards at all. The ad provided little information about the product itself, but had a lot to say about the miracles it could perform for people with diabetes, high cholesterol, and prostate issues. Its Web site did not list the product's ingredients, or any research studies to back up the claims that the advertisers made. I gave it a thumbs-down, told Karen to save her money, and thanked her for consulting me.

Health information is everywhere—in newspapers, magazines, books, television, the Internet, billboards, on food packages, at the health food store, even from well-meaning friends and loved ones. How can you tell if it is reliable?

IN THIS CHAPTER, YOU WILL:

- Learn how to find reliable information from a variety of media sources.
- Review a list of recommended Web sites.
- Learn how to determine if a health-care professional is qualified.
- Discover ways to encourage your health-care team to provide you with the information and support that you desire.
- Make another Jump-Start Pledge.

STEP 9

Check Your Information

NEWSPAPERS—FACT OR FICTION?

NEWSPAPERS ARE NOTORIOUS for misquoting. It is all about speed. In the newspaper world, time is of the essence. When a story breaks, reporters rush to get details and send the story on its way. Be wary of facts found in hurriedly reported stories of breakthroughs and cures, or longtime medical practices that are suddenly condemned. In-depth exposés prepared by expert columnists are generally written with more care; these journalists usually have adequate time to examine and confirm their facts. Quality articles should reveal the sources of their information—a research center, government agency, respected organization or university, or known experts with appropriate credentials.

Fortunately, we have a tremendous diabetes advocate in a high-level decision-making role. Fran Carpentier is the senior editor of *Parade*, the national Sunday newspaper magazine. Fran has type 1 diabetes and passionately encourages her magazine to showcase many well-researched, diabetes-related stories:

I am the person who is always suggesting that we need to do another diabetes story. I'm the one who suggested very passionately . . . that we should do a very level-headed piece on stem cell research, which of course is very controversial right now, and I was thrilled when the idea was embraced . . . I'm sort of the poster child of diabetes. I also take a great interest in any other health stories we do, because really and truly, most of the major health problems that we have . . . really have to do with diabetes, because a lot of heart disease and strokes are the results of people having uncontrolled diabetes . . . I don't think that I've made everyone crazy yet, but they know that they've got a very strong proponent for giving the American people as much and as up-to-date information as they should have.

MAGAZINES

MANY MAGAZINES DO a nice job of checking their facts. Unlike newspapers that demand immediate news updates, magazine articles are written several weeks to months in advance. Thorough research can be done and qualified reviewers have time to confirm the facts.

Open a diabetes magazine and glance through its first few pages. Do you see a list of editorial board members? These are the folks who approve article choices and review them for accuracy. As with the experts quoted in newspapers, editorial board member should have recognized medical credentials, and ideally be associated with a research center, university, health organization, or government agency, or be known experts in the field. If the qualifications of these board members seem questionable, the advice found in the articles may be questionable as well.

Christine Gorman, senior health writer at *Time* magazine, shares her own thoughts about the information that is available today:

Particularly now, with the Internet, there's so much information out there that is of a very different quality . . . It's very easy to be seduced by a story that sounds good, that makes sense. We are storytelling people . . . There are some great stories and there are a lot of believable stories . . . Part of what we're trying to do in medicine now, I think, is to make things evidence based. Can you prove it? Is it more than just a good story? . . . Being a little skeptical is always good. Looking for proof—is this just one person who is saying this or is it several different labs? Science goes by what has been replicated. Can other people do it? Can other people get the same results? . . . Who is the source of the information? Has it been replicated? Have other people come up with the same answers? Is there consensus about it? . . . In medicine, things tend to move forward by consensus . . . A lot of times when many people are agreed on something, you really need to pay attention to that. If somebody is saying that "They are all wet," [that person needs] to have some pretty compelling evidence.

INTERNET RESOURCES

THE INTERNET IS a jungle filled with thousands of diabetes-related and health Web sites. Some are helpful and accurate, and others less so. Many want you to purchase products, but use unqualified "experts" and anecdotal quotes from supposedly satisfied customers to promote them. Sadly, no monitoring organization exists to check Web sites for medical accuracy. You may occasionally find award logos posted on some sites, but these are given for excellence in design and service, not for data reliability.

Search for sites that are affiliated with recognized organizations or individuals, as mentioned above.

Here are a few Web sites that provide reliable i

- *Americanheart.org*—the site of the American He
- *Angelarose.com/famousdiabetics*—a list of fa with diabetes
- *Caloriecontrol.org*—Web site of the Calorie Control Council. Offers information about sweeteners and other weight-loss products
- *Calorieking.com*—offers nutrient information
- *Centerwatch.com*—provides lists of medical research studies that you can participate in
- *Childrenwithdiabetes.com*
- *Consumerlab.com*—an independent site that reviews the safety and effectiveness of herbs and supplements
- *Diabeteseducator.org*
- *Diabetes.niddk.nih.gov*—site of the National Diabetes Information Clearinghouse, run by the National Institute of Diabetes and Digestive and Kidney Diseases and National Institutes of Health (NIH)
- *Siabetes.org*—American Diabetes Association
- *Diabetesmonitor.com*
- *dLife.com*—affiliated with the *dLifeTV* weekly television program on CNBC
- *Drinet.org*—Diabetes Research Institute
- *Eatright.org*—American Dietetic Association
- *Healthfinder.gov*—run by the U.S. Department of Health and Human Services; provides a list of reliable Web sites
- *Idf.org*—The International Diabetes Federation
- *Intellihealth.com*—consumer medical information from Harvard Medical School
- *Jdrf.org*—Juvenile Diabetes Association; contains detailed research updates
- *Joslin.org*—Joslin Diabetes Center

- *Medlineplus.gov*—provides information about medications and medical conditions. Sponsored by the U.S. National Library of Medicine and NIH
- *Mendosa.com/diabetes.htm*—diabetes directory
- *Quackwatch.com*—provides a guide to medical misinformation and health fraud; check out Internet rumors at this site
- *Snopes.com*—debunks Internet rumors
- *Urbanlegends.about.com*—debunks Internet rumors
- *Webmd.com*—a source of reliable medical information on numerous topics

I also invite you to visit my personal Web site, dearjanis.com, for articles, informative newsletters, warm and caring interactive support on the monitored message board, and informative interview highlights from my weekly radio program.

Few bulletin boards, chat rooms, or blogs are monitored by health professionals. Several that are include joslin.org, dlife.com, dearjanis.com, and TCOYD.com. But even when policed well, it may take a day or two before a suspicious comment is corrected or deleted. Check out all medical information that you find with your health-care team or at quackwatch.com. To find out if a rumor is valid, visit urbandlegends.about.com, snopes.com, or any other urban legend buster.

Bulletin boards and chat rooms offer opportunities to connect with others who have diabetes, and can introduce you to new ideas that you may want to explore further. A recent study conducted by the Joslin Diabetes Center in Boston found that nearly 75 percent of those interviewed felt that the Internet boards helped them cope with their diabetes. Seventy-one percent said that they helped them feel more hopeful.

BOOKS

UNLIKE AN INTERNET site, you can toss a book into a purse or bag and read it wherever you go, dog-ear your favorite pages, and underline interesting comments. Books are a terrific source for information that has been checked, reviewed, and reviewed again. The only downside is that many books take some time to go from conception to actual publication, so the information may be a bit outdated. Check the copyright page for how recently a book has been published or updated; and also look at a few pages to see how in-depth, clear, and user-friendly the writing is. Note the author's credentials, as mentioned earlier, and be wary of self-published works that are written by an author whose only qualification is that he or she has diabetes. These tales may be inspirational, but are often filled with inaccurate or even dangerous suggestions. And remember, a best-seller may or may not contain advice that is appropriate for you. You still need to view all that you read with a critical eye.

TELEVISION

LEARNING HAS NEVER been more convenient. With a click of the remote, and a bit of help from your TiVo program recorder, you can enjoy health programs at any time of the day or night. But is the information honest and reliable? It depends. In-depth magazine-type programs such as *60 Minutes* and *20/20* are generally well planned and reviewed. A weekly show such as *dLifeTV* on CNBC has its programming rigorously reviewed by a qualified medical staff. Breaking news reports, on the other hand, can be misleading. Stories about medical cures and breakthroughs are often rushed onto the air before they have been examined by the medical community for accuracy and reliability.

Disregard infomercials. These are commercials that are disguised as regular programs. They generally offer biased information with one purpose only—to entice you to purchase a product. Some are easy to spot. Think of all the cutlery demonstrations you've watched over the years. The salesperson stares right at you through the camera and emphatically invites you to rush to the phone, with your credit card in hand, to purchase an item that you apparently can't live without. "It slices . . . it dices!" "You must have this!"

Another type of infomercial is less obvious and far more devious. It appears to be a legitimate interview in which an "expert" sits at a table and discusses a medical topic with an enthusiastic host. The expert subtly drops hints about his product and its benefits. He or she may claim to have a cure that is being ignored by the mainstream medical community or has uncovered an ancient treatment that no one knows about. It is a very soft-sell that can hook you in, if you let it. If a conversation repeatedly refers to a particular product that a person has developed, you are watching an infomercial.

UNDERSTANDING CREDENTIALS

AFTER YOU'VE GATHERED your information from the media, seek input from a qualified health-care professional. Some will have a "CDE" or "BC-ADM" after their name. CDE means they are a certified diabetes educator, and BC-ADM, a board-certified advanced diabetes manager. The CDE can be earned by many health professionals including physicians, clinical psychologists, registered nurses, occupational therapists, physical therapists, registered dietitians, podiatrists, optometrists, and pharmacists. These individuals have completed a required amount of patient care hours, passed a comprehensive written exam, participate in continuing education opportunities and are recognized by the American Association of Diabetes Educators. The BC-ADM is an advanced diabetes credential that can be earned by registered nurses, dietitians, and pharmacists. All should be able to provide you with information that you can trust. To learn more about certified diabetes educators or to locate one in your area, visit diabeteseducator.org.

Be wary of those who call themselves specialists, yet have no expertise in that field. For example, the term "nutritionist" is not legally protected and can be used by anyone regardless of the amount of knowledge that he or she has.

STEP 10
Be a Partner in Your Diabetes Care

ABBY, one of my patients, was recently diagnosed with type 2 diabetes. While visiting a popular diabetes Web site, she learned about a new type of insulin that everyone seemed to be using. She wanted to try it, too, but wasn't sure if she should. When she asked her doctor about it, he curtly told her that if she wasn't happy with his care, she should go elsewhere. His response was a total surprise.

SOME HEALTH-CARE providers are reluctant to have patients take charge of their diabetes. It goes contrary to how these specialists have been taught. During training, they learn to assess problems and solve them. That works fine in a crisis, such as treating a broken arm or a heart attack, but daily diabetes care is different.

They might have a standard approach to whoever walks in with diabetes, ignoring that their patients have individual needs, because it is easier for them to do so: your doctor may automatically prescribe insulin syringes, not knowing that you prefer insulin pens instead, because you frequently inject out in public, at meetings, and in restaurants. Your dietitian may teach you to count carbohydrates, but you prefer to use a method that doesn't require any counting at all, such as the Plate Method. But it is you who lives with your diabetes day in and day out, and should have a voice in your care plan. The more input that you have in your medical and lifestyle decisions, the more motivated you will be to follow whatever regimen is proposed. The act of turning control over to a patient has a name—it is called the Empowerment Approach.

THE EMPOWERMENT APPROACH

AFTER WORKING IN the field of diabetes for many years, diabetes educators Bob Anderson and Martha Funnell found that the best outcomes occurred when patients played a decision-making role in how their disease should be treated. To teach this, they designed the Empowerment Approach—a strategy that puts you, the patient, in the driver's seat and encourages your health-care team to be the support system. If you aren't in that role, make every effort to get there. During an interview about the Empowerment Approach, Martha Funnell responded to the following two questions:

Did you receive a lot of resistance from health-care professionals to this new approach?

Initially, we did. People were very hesitant, because they were concerned that people with diabetes would not accept the amount of responsibility that they felt was needed in order to manage this very complex disease. But the reality was that people with diabetes had been doing that all along . . . people with diabetes are in charge.

What are a patient's responsibilities?

First of all, I think it's important to understand that it is in fact a shared responsibility. That we need to be collaborators with our providers, because once you're out of the doctor's office or the nurse practitioner's office or even the education program, you go home to make decisions each and every day about what's going to happen, and those decisions are what determine your future with diabetes. So you really need the expertise of the health professional. But their role is then to serve as your coach, and your guide, and your teacher. One of the first things to do is to learn all that you can, because to be an effective collaborator, you need to know what it is that you need to collaborate about—what's important for you and also what decisions you make [and] what the potential outcomes are.

YOUR HEALTH-CARE TEAM:
- Your primary physician
- Your endocrinologist or diabetologist
- Your registered dietitian, preferably a CDE
- Your diabetes educator, preferably a CDE
- Your eye doctor—ophthalmologist
- Your foot doctor—podiatrist
- Your pharmacist
- Your mental health care professional—social worker or counselor

Search for health-care providers who are open to you and your needs. If you don't feel comfortable speaking with a particular specialist, find another. Don't keep your health-care choices a secret from those who advise you. If you feel you need to hide treatment behaviors from your team, such as herb and supplement use or acupuncture, then you must search for team members with whom you can talk openly.

MEMBERS OF YOUR HEALTH-CARE TEAM SHOULD:
- Respect your opinion
- Be open to the information that you bring
- Focus on you when you are together
- Offer reliable and safe treatment choices
- Help motivate you to improve

THEY SHOULD NOT:
- Automatically dismiss the information that you wish to share
- Insult you when you fail
- Threaten you when your control is less than perfect

A counseling approach that puts you in control demands more from your team than many of your specialists are used to giving. It takes more time to discuss a choice than to verbalize a direct order or write out a prescription. As you can imagine, this new approach can be tough. Is your team up to the challenge?

EVALUATE YOUR CURRENT TEAM:

They listen to my concerns.	YES	NO
They are open to new ideas.	YES	NO
They encourage me.	YES	NO
They know what is new in diabetes.	YES	NO

If you've answered no to any of the above statements, take action. Request a greater role in the decision-making process and ask for additional conversation time. If your provider is not receptive, find a different one.

The best type of specialist to see when you have diabetes is an endocrinologist—an expert in diabetes and other hormonal issues. Most family physicians and internists don't have time to keep up-to-date with the new developments in diabetes, but an endocrinologist does. Ask your primary care doctor or another member of your health-care team to recommend an endocrinologist whom he or she respects, or get a referral from aace.com, the official site of the American Association of Clinical Endocrinologists. If your request is met with a less-than-enthusiastic response, don't let that deter you. This is your diabetes and you deserve the best treatment available. If your physician is unwilling to share your care with a specialist, or who takes it as a personal criticism, perhaps it is time to find another physician who puts your needs first.

Your other supporting team members should be well versed in diabetes also. If you are not receiving the most qualified advice, find a different specialist. Ask for a recommendation from your endocrinologist, local hospital, or a friend who also has diabetes. Visit diabeteseducator.org to locate a nearby certified diabetes educator, attend a diabetes class at your local hospital, or seek support from reliable Web sites.

A Helpful Tool

The AADE-7 Self-Care Behaviors worksheet is one way to be sure that you get the advice that you need from all of your team members. Designed by the American Association of Diabetes Educators, these seven self-care behavior topics are:

- Healthy eating
- Being active
- Monitoring
- Taking medication
- Problem solving
- Healthy coping
- Reducing risks

Set a personal goal within your chosen topic with the guidance of your diabetes educator. For example, under the topic of "Healthy Eating," you can choose one of the following options to work on until your next visit:

- Make at least some food choices that are discussed during your visit.
- Reduce your portion sizes of all of the foods that you eat.
- Follow a specific meal plan designed during the visit.
- Create your own personalized goal.

The beauty of this worksheet is that it helps other educators reinforce personal diabetes goals that you have already chosen and helps keep you on track. Each sheet comes in multiple copies. After it is filled out with your behavior preferences and choice of actions, you receive a copy to take home and another copy stays in your medical file for future use. Whoever opens your file will know what tasks you have chosen, what guidance you have already received, and your own assessment of your progress. He or she can move on from there, and keep you in charge of your progress. These sheets are available from diabeteseducator.org, the official Web site of the American Association of Diabetes Educators.

Organizing Your Priorities

Now that your team is assembled, here are some ways to get the most out of each visit:

- Before your visit, jot down topics that you'd like to discuss with your health-care team, including personal issues such as sexual problems. Your doctor may not ask about these issues, so you must bring them up.
- If possible, get any required lab tests run prior to your appointment, so they can be discussed during your visit.
- Review your blood glucose results. Highlight the highs and lows with a bright marker so that you and your team can spot patterns and areas of concern.
- List herbs, minerals, supplements, or over-the-counter medications that you would like to take. Some interfere with other medications and may alter the recommendations that your team makes regarding your care.
- Bring articles that you wish to discuss.
- Ask that your diabetes care goals be written on an AADE-7 worksheet, or into your medical file.

You are the head of your diabetes care team, and all of your health goals should be chosen by you, based on knowledge that you've discovered combined with reliable advice and guidance that you've gleaned from the experts on your team. You don't have to continue to work with team members who don't support your goals.

CHOOSE YOUR JUMP-START PLEDGE

- I pledge to choose an action from the AADE7 worksheet and do it for one week.
- I pledge to expand my knowledge of diabetes and read a few minutes from a book or reliable Web site every day for one week.
- I pledge to discuss with my health-care team a new treatment option I would like to try.
- I pledge to add to my health-care team an additional member who is qualified to help me with special issues.
- I pledge to [your choice] for one week.

TAKE CHARGE

Enlist the help of experts who will listen to you. You should be able to discuss with your health-care team any of your concerns and any treatments that you wish to try.

6

SAY YES TO...
Enjoying the Foods You Love

> If I had to live by a half an apple, a baked chicken wing, and iceberg lettuce, every day & forever, I would have a big problem with my doctor. I will not allow my diabetes to take away my freedom to enjoy real food. I'd rather listen to my body, to make better food choices, and necessary adjustments.
>
> —from "Yogiraj,"
> on the dearjanis.com message board

D**O YOU FEEL** guilty when you eat certain foods? You're not alone. Many people feel guilty when they eat foods that they know will send their blood sugar level soaring or cause their weight to climb, such as a slice of wedding cake or a chocolate bar. But you *can* eat the things you love. Here's how to fit your favorite treats back into your life.

IN THIS CHAPTER, YOU WILL:

- Learn why you may desire certain foods.
- Discover ways to transform favorite recipes into healthier versions.
- Examine popular sugar substitutes.
- Review successful grocery shopping tips.
- Make a Jump-Start Pledge.

STEP 11

Examine Why You Desire Certain Foods

SOME PEOPLE BELIEVE that eating the foods they love, in reasonable portions, can be done without compromising their diabetes control; it helps them enjoy life and feel less deprived. Others feel that a strict change in dietary choices is a small price to pay for optimal control. As Howard Steinberg, the founder and CEO of *dLifeTV*, likes to say, "It's the law of small numbers—less insulin, less eating, less mistakes." The choice is entirely up to you.

Before you learn how to include forbidden foods in your diabetic meal plan, ponder this question: Do you really want a particular food, or are you being convinced to want it by slick marketing campaigns? Dr. Brian Wansink, head of the Cornell University Food and Brand Lab, studies the marketing forces that push us to yearn for certain foods and eat them in larger portions than we probably should. The lab consists of fifteen researchers and three test kitchens, with five cooperating supermarkets, and a panel of three thousand consumers. Here are some of the studies that his team ran, and the lessons they learned:

- *How food is described will increase your desire for it*—Does even just the name of an item affect the amount that we choose to eat? A study of cafeteria patrons showed that a dessert marked "Grandma's Homemade Apple Pie" enjoyed greater sales than a similar item with a less nostalgic name. In another study, two groups were given identical bottles of wine at a dinner that displayed different labels. One claimed to be from California, a state known for its superb wines, and the other from North Dakota. Those who received the California wine enjoyed it thoroughly. In fact, they raved about the entire meal. The group with the North Dakota wine drank little of it, and voiced complaints about both the wine and the meal.

- *The size of the package affects the amount you consume*—The research team separated a number of participants into two separate groups. One received a package of M&M's candies that contained 114 pieces, and the other was given a bag with three times that amount. Those with the smaller package ate about 63 pieces, for an average of 209 calories. Those who had the larger bag ate an average of 103 candies, for a grand total of 341 calories.

  On another occasion, free popcorn was passed out to a group of movie-goers. Some received a large container, and the others were given an extra-large portion. Regardless of their hunger, those who had the extra-large container ate 44 percent more than those with the smaller bag. According to Wansink, when food comes in a larger package, we don't try to conserve, so we eat more. (An extra fact—people eat 15 percent more popcorn while watching a sad movie!)

- *A food's location affects the amount that you eat*—Dr. Wansink's team placed thirty Hershey's Kisses into two types of candy dishes—one clear and the other opaque. Several were placed on top of a secretary's desk, and others were placed six feet away from the desk. As expected, more pieces were taken from the dishes on the desk that displayed their contents visibly; the less visible and less

convenient the food item, the lower the temptation. If you want to eat less of a certain food, hide it far away. If you wish to encourage yourself and others to consume healthier foods, such as cut-up vegetables, place them within easy reach in a container that makes them visibly inviting.
- *Your familiarity with a food affects the amount that you eat—* To explore this, the team compared the eating behavior of people who put olive oil on their bread with those who used butter. The olive-oil eaters ate less bread. Olive oil may be more satisfying than butter, but is also less familiar. It is apparently easier to eat greater amounts of a familiar food than of an unfamiliar one. We are also drawn to foods that connect us to happier times and Mom's love. Men prefer hearty and savory foods, such as steak, pasta, pizza, and casseroles; women prefer snacks, chocolate, and candy. The most popular American comfort food of all is potato chips.

There are, of course, additional reasons why you may want to eat certain foods as Maggie Powers explains in *Forbidden Foods Diabetic Cooking:*

> Many foods are part of our personal history and have followed us on our journey through life . . . Because of these experiences we like to have certain foods at holidays, birthdays, and other celebrations. Special foods are part of our traditions, traditions we want to maintain and pass on to others. Many of us have favorite recipes we want to share with our family and friends. Just because you have diabetes, you don't want to give up this part of who you are—and you don't have to!

Food plays a significant role in our lives, which is why it is so difficult to adhere to a regimen that removes beloved foods from the table. Here are some ways to alter your favorite recipes and food choices so they fit comfortably into your diabetic meal plan.

READJUST YOUR FAVORITE FOODS

TODAY'S NEWER MEDICATIONS, designer insulin, insulin pumps, and improved care, enable you to eat almost any food, in a reasonable amount. But not every choice is a wise one. Some contain unhealthy amounts of cholesterol or trans fats, or have a carbohydrate content that requires you to take higher amounts of insulin than you might want to use. With a few small adjustments, you can transform many of your favorite foods into healthier versions. The following is an example by Chef Michel Nischan, author of *Taste—Pure And Simple* and *Homegrown—Pure And Simple*:

• CHICKEN FLORENTINE •
(Michel's original version)

SERVES 6

¾ cup dry bread crumbs
¼ cup Parmesan cheese
3 whole chicken breasts, skinned, boned, and split
½ cup sliced green onions
2 tablespoons butter
2 tablespoons flour
1 cup milk
1 (10-ounce) package frozen chopped spinach, thawed

Preheat the oven to 350°F. Combine the bread crumbs and cheese. Dip the chicken breast halves in the crumb mixture to coat lightly. Arrange in a baking dish. In a saucepan, cook the onion in the butter until tender. Blend in the flour. Stir in the milk all at once. Cook, stirring, until thick and bubbly. Cook and stir for 1 minute more. Stir in the spinach. Spoon the spinach mixture over chicken and sprinkle with rest of crumb mixture. Bake, uncovered, at 350° F for 40 to 45 minutes.

NUTRIENT CONTENT PER SERVING:
249 calories; 8.65 g fat; 16.4 g carb; 26 g protein

• CHICKEN FLORENTINE •
(Michel's healthier version)

SERVES 6

- ¼ cup lightly crushed flaxseeds
- ¼ cup lightly crushed mustard seeds
- ¼ cup ground almonds
- 3 whole chicken breasts, skinned, boned, and split
- ½ cup sliced green onions
- 1 tablespoon grape seed oil
- ¼ cup chicken broth
- ½ cup low-fat sour cream
- ¼ cup low-fat Parmesan cheese
- 1 (10-ounce) package frozen chopped spinach, thawed and well drained

Preheat the oven to 350°F. Thoroughly combine the flaxseeds, mustard seeds, and crushed almonds. Dip the chicken breast halves in the mixture to coat lightly. Arrange in a baking dish. In a saucepan, cook the onion in the grape seed oil until tender. Add the well-drained spinach and cook, stirring constantly, for 2 to 3 minutes, until the spinach begins to heat through. Add the chicken broth and sour cream. Stir in the Parmesan until well combined. Spoon the spinach mixture over the chicken, and sprinkle with the rest of the mixture. Bake, uncovered, at 350° F for 40 to 45 minutes.

NUTRIENT CONTENT PER SERVING:
267 calories; 11.23 g fat; 13.3 g carb; 29.1 g protein

Both of these delicious recipes have similar nutrient contents, but vary in their health benefits. The first version uses butter and whole milk, which are high in cholesterol. The improved version incorporates heart-healthy ingredients—almonds, flaxseeds, and grape seed oil. Michel also substitutes low-fat sour cream for the milk, which offers additional flavor without the fat. A healthier recipe never has to compromise on taste.

YOU CAN MAKE THE CHANGE

THE TRANSITION TO healthier eating is worthwhile but can be a challenge, especially if family members expect certain foods to appear on the table. When Mother Love, one of the hosts of *dLifeTV* who has type 2 diabetes, started transforming her family's favorite recipes into diabetes-friendly and heart-healthy versions, her son protested. Fortunately, her husband became her biggest supporter and helped her explain this new cuisine transition to their son. Mother Love reports that he said:

> "Your mother has diabetes. We will have to help her manage diabetes. We don't have it and we're not going to get it, but she's not a short order cook." 'Cause my son protested . . ."Oh, Ma, why do I have to eat twigs, sprigs, sprouts, and leaves? I'm a growing guy. I'm only twelve. Why can't I eat this, why can't I eat that? I want a real hamburger."

But Mother Love didn't give up. She knew that she could successfully prepare foods in a healthier way . . . as long as her son didn't see the tricks that she was playing.

> He was off of ground beef for two years before he realized that I was fixing him ground turkey. You know, with guys, if you

just hide the boxes and labels, they never even know, they don't even know!

Here are some suggestions that can help you enjoy many of your favorite foods in a healthier way:

1. *Cut your portion size*
    - Use a smaller plate at mealtime.
    - Don't take your own piece of dessert; take a taste from a friend's dish.
    - When at a buffet, choose your foods then quickly move away from the table.

2. *Use artificial sweeteners*—Noncalorie sugar substitutes, such as Splenda, Equal, and Sweet 'N Low, can help you reduce the carbohydrate and calorie content of many different foods. If you are concerned about their safety, the research is overwhelmingly positive, but the decision is ultimately up to you. These sugar substitutes have been tested repeatedly in numerous countries and are well tolerated by most people. Here is some information about each specific sweetener:
    - *Acesulfame K*—Sold under the name of Sweet One and Sunette, this product is a concentrated sweetener that is 200 times sweeter than sugar. It is very stable in heat so it can be used in all types of baked products and recipes. It is also found in commercial products such as candy, drinks, and chewing gum. The Web site for this product is sweetone.com.
    - *Saccharin*—Saccharin is 300 times sweeter than sugar. It is sold as Sweet 'N Low and Sugar Twin, and performs well in both hot and cold dishes. Some people find that it has a slight aftertaste, but it loses it when combined with other sweeteners. In the midseventies, FDA

banned saccharin from the market after learning that it could cause cancer in rats. Additional research, however, found that the sweetener was not the culprit, but the rats themselves—they had a predisposition to developing cancer, so in December 2000, President Clinton signed legislation that removed its warning label and the controversy ended. See sweetnlow.com for additional information and recipes.

- *Aspartame*—Sold as NutraSweet and Equal, this sweetener has been the subject of numerous false Internet rumors. The truth is that most people can enjoy it without difficulty, but it should be avoided by individuals who have the rare disease penylketonuria (PKU), as they are unable to metabolize phenylalanine, one of its main ingredients. Those who experience headaches or dizziness when using it should avoid it also. It can be used in most recipes, but may lose some of its sweetness if subjected to prolonged heating. When preparing an item on a stovetop, add this sweetener after you remove the item from the heat. The blue packets of Equal are highly concentrated—200 times sweeter than sugar. A less concentrated version, Equal Spoonful, can be used cup for cup to replace sugar. Baking and cooking and measuring guidelines are available at equal.com.
- *Sucralose*—Marketed as Splenda, sucralose is made from sugar, but is an artificial sweetener. It is created when three hydroxyl groups on the sugar molecule are replaced by three atoms of chlorine. The granular form can be used in recipes in which sugar provides sweetness, such as pies, cookies, marinades, glazes, and muffins—the granular Splenda replaces the equivalent quantity of sugar. Splenda's sugar/sucralose mixture, however, is recommended for baked goods in which sugar does more than supply sweetness; it

assists with the browning, volume and moistness of the product. Use a half cup of that in place of an entire cup of sugar. For additional information, visit splenda.com.
- *Stevia*—Stevia is a natural, calorie-free sweetener that is 100 to 300 times sweeter than sugar. It is plant-derived and has been used in teas and other foods for years in Paraguay; it was developed into a zero-calorie sweetener in Japan in the 1970s. When taken in excessively high doses (250 to 500 mg, three times a day) it may reduce blood pressure levels. This amount is significantly larger than any person is likely to use, but it shows that stevia may have some unknown effect on the cardiovascular system. More U.S. studies must be done before the FDA will approve stevia as a sugar substitute. Any item that receives FDA approval must be able to be used in generous quantities by a wide variety of individuals. The stevia Web site is stevia.com.

3. *Limit your fats*—Reduce the amount of fat in a recipe as much as possible without compromising the quality of the dish.
    - Use low-fat or reduced-fat versions of regular cheese, deli meats, and salad dressings.
    - Use a nonstick cooking spray.
    - Substitute evaporated skim milk for heavy cream.
    - Replace sour cream with fat-free sour cream or plain yogurt.
    - Use skim or 1% milk.
    - Use less cheese. Stronger-flavored cheeses such as blue, Parmesan, Romano, and Cheddar can be used in reduced amounts to add flavor.
    - Substitute sherbet, low-fat ice cream, or frozen yogurt for regular ice cream.

- Enjoy baked versions of snacks foods, such as baked tortilla and potato chips, in place of fried ones. Choose those that are also trans fat free.
- A bagel can be used in place of a croissant.
- Place your salad dressing on the side and touch your fork to it before dipping into your salad. You will enjoy a taste of dressing in every bite and limit your intake.
- An egg's fat is in its yolk. Use two egg whites to replace a single whole egg in a recipe, or use an egg-substitute products available at your local grocery.
- Prepare soups, stews, meatballs, and so on ahead of time, and chill. Remove the fat before reheating.
- Grill, bake, and broil instead of frying.
- Remove the skin from chicken prior to cooking. Cover with a sauce or seal tightly with foil wrap to help keep it moist.
- Try Enova brand oil in place of other vegetable oils. Enova is a newly designed oil product that is not used by the body in the same way as other oils. The shape of certain molecules in Enova makes it more difficult for the body to store it as fat. Foods prepared with this new oil taste the same as those made with other vegetable oils.

4. *Reduce your salt*—As mentioned earlier, not everyone needs to cut back on their sodium intake, but experts do believe that an excessive intake of sodium can encourage the development of high blood pressure. If you have been instructed to limit your sodium intake, or just wish to cut back a bit, try the following:
    - Use salt-free seasonings in place of table salt.
    - Experiment with natural flavorings such as fresh herbs, lemon, lime and orange juices, pepper, onion, and garlic.

- Buy low-sodium canned soups, gravies, bouillon mixes, and tomato and vegetable products.
- Limit your intake of prepared and fast-food food items. Many contain generous amounts of sodium.
- Taste your food *before* salting it. You may need to add less or none at all.

5. *Increase your fiber*—There are two types of fiber: soluble, which helps lower blood cholesterol, and insoluble, which helps maintain healthy bowel function. Increasing your intake of both is helpful. High-soluble fiber foods include oatmeal, oat bran, beans, barley peas, rice bran, citrus fruits, and strawberries. Insoluble-fiber-containing foods include whole-grain cereals, whole-grain bread, wheat bran, barley, rye, beets, Brussels sprouts, cauliflower, cabbage, and turnips.
    - Replace white rice, processed bread, and regular noodles with whole-grain versions.
    - Substitute whole wheat flour and whole wheat pastry flour for a portion of the white flour in your recipes. If you substitute the entire amount, you may end up with a heavy, less appealing product.
    - Sprinkle uncooked quick oatmeal into meatballs, meatloaf, and other similar dishes.
    - Add low-fat granola to yogurt or low-fat ice cream.
    - Choose cereals that are higher in fiber.
    - Sprinkle wheat bran or ground flaxseeds onto your breakfast cereal.

6. *Lower the blood-sugar-raising effect of your food*
    - Take smaller portions.
    - Use lower-carbohydrate versions of breads, yogurt, milk, and other foods.
    - Eat your food with a well-balanced meal that contains protein and some fat.

- Choose foods that have a lower glycemic index value, as discussed in chapter 2.
- Increase the fiber content of the meal.
- Take a walk or do some light physical activity after eating.
- Drink plenty of water—this helps lower blood sugar levels once they have become elevated.
- Take additional insulin or oral medication (with the approval of your health-care team).

STEP 12

Shop Wisely

A VISIT TO your local grocery store may be overwhelming, especially if you try to cook differently for the rest of your family. Even though you may be the only one who has diabetes, you can prepare diabetes-friendly meals for all members of your family. Don't make two shopping lists or prepare two different entrées each night. The changes that you make to your recipes are appropriate and healthy for your entire family. Here are a few suggestions to help you enjoy a successful shopping trip:

- Review your meal plan and write down the foods that you need for the week.
- Don't shop while hungry. You will be less likely to make impulse purchases.
- If your schedule is hectic, choose ready-made salads and vegetable sticks. But be prepared to pay a bit more.
- Watch out for foods that make specific nutritional claims:
    - Low-sugar and low-fat foods may not be low in calories.
    - Low-fat foods may be high in sugar or sodium.
    - Low-sugar foods may be high in fat.

- Beware of the word "dietetic." It refers to any food that has been prepared for a special diet—not necessarily a diabetic one.
- Don't purchase foods that you prefer not to eat. If a family member is a huge ice-cream fan and you want to stay away from it, don't buy any. Your loved one can always head out to an ice-cream parlor for a special treat.
- Have fun and purchase some "free foods." Two to three servings of foods with less than 20 calories or less than 5 grams of carbohydrate per serving can usually be eaten at intervals during the day without experiencing a rise in blood sugar.

Turn your shopping adventure into an exercise workout by pushing your cart up and down all of the aisles in the store, even if you have no interest in a particular section. Do you wear a pedometer (a step counter)? If you do, it will make this suggestion even more enjoyable. Pedometers are relatively inexpensive and can be purchased from athletic stores, discount stores, and pharmacies. To start, wear your new pedometer for one week without altering your activity level. When the week ends, divide your step total by seven to determine your daily step average. Now the fun begins. Each day, try to beat that total by 1,000 steps. It sounds like a lot, but you will see that it takes very little additional effort to do it.

KEEP GRANDMA'S RECIPES ALIVE

DO YOU HAVE favorite family recipes that have been passed down from generation to generation? The recipes that you loved can be enjoyed again with a few simple changes. Use the suggestions listed above to create healthier versions of family favorites.

CHOOSE YOUR JUMP-START PLEDGE

- I pledge to add one whole-grain food to my diet each day of this week.
- I pledge to add one extra serving of colorful or dark vegetables to my diet each day this week.
- I pledge to replace one fast-food/prepared meal with a homemade one, one day this week.
- I pledge to prepare one family recipe in a healthier way this week.
- I pledge to taste my food before I salt it for one week.
- I pledge to eat my dinner off of a smaller plate for one week.
- I pledge to [your choice] for one week.

TAKE CHARGE

EAT HEALTHIER VERSIONS OF THE FOODS YOU LOVE.

7

SAY YES TO...
An Active Social Life

I HAVE MET numerous patients who feel so trapped by their diabetes that they rarely socialize with friends or family anymore. They shy away from workplace celebrations and rarely attend family dinners. Diabetes doesn't have to interfere with your social life. I'd like to share some ways for you to enjoy your social engagements at work, with family, and with friends, with minimal diabetes interference.

IN THIS CHAPTER, YOU WILL:

- Learn how to keep your diabetes from interfering with social events at the office.
- Keep your diabetes from becoming a problem when out with friends.
- Help prevent your diabetes from becoming a challenge while on a date.
- Explore ways to stop diabetes from interfering with your sex life.

- Learn treatment options that you can use if you experience sexual complications.
- Add another Jump-Start Pledge.

STEP 13
Plan Ahead When You Socialize

AT YOUR OFFICE

DAVE, *a friend of mine, was working at his desk when his co-workers brought out a cake to celebrate the birthday of one of his fellow sales reps. He was prepared to head over to the party and grab a diet beverage when he remembered that he had his glucose monitor in his briefcase. He checked his blood sugar level and found that it was on the low end of his normal range. He could easily enjoy a small piece of cake. A 2-inch slice of unfrosted cake has about 17 grams of carbohydrate and a frosted slice of the same size contains about 30 grams. From experience, he knew that he could handle that amount. If his glucose started to run a bit high in a few hours, he knew what he could do—drink some water, take a brisk walk, and delay his next meal for a brief period of time.*

Keep your glucose meter handy—at your office, or in your purse or briefcase—so you can test wherever you are and make choices that meet your needs. Years ago, people with diabetes didn't have access to glucose monitors and used guesswork to plan their next move. You have this technology, so use it to have your cake and eat it, too.

TESTING AND INJECTIONS

CAN YOU CHECK your blood and inject insulin in public? Yes, both can be done discreetly.

It is now very easy to monitor your blood glucose level while you are out or among other people. Your glucose monitor comes with a carrying case that opens easily across your lap. If you normally test with your materials spread across a table, practice doing it on your lap. It may feel awkward at first, but the more you do it, the more agile you will become. This will free you up to check your blood quickly at any location. Or you can do what Matthew, a friend of mine, does, and enlist the help of a friend: "At intermissions of performances, I'll usually ask a friend, if I'm with one, to spread his or her palm, on which I'll rest my kit, and use it to test. Every friend I've ever asked to do this is very happy to help." Or, if you wish for more privacy, excuse yourself and go to a restroom.

You can inject insulin right through your clothing. The most covert way to do this is with an insulin pen. This method works best with darker clothes, as occasionally a droplet of blood may appear on your skin and stain your clothing.

You Can Mix Food and Business

Business meetings and get-togethers can be stressful for anyone. Add diabetes, food, and possibly alcohol, and you could be headed for trouble. If you are invited for a meal, request a copy of the restaurant's menu ahead of time; most establishments will fax a copy to your office. It is easier to plan meal choices when there are few distractions. Restaurants usually honor special food requests, so ask for an item to be baked or broiled instead of fried, or request that a sauce or salad dressing be omitted or placed on the side. If the menu is limited, eat before you go and enjoy a beverage, bowl of vegetable soup, or simple salad as your friends eat their meals.

Keep a supply of peanut butter, rice cakes, crackers, juice boxes, dried fruit, granola bars, nuts, diabetes-friendly meal replacement drinks and bars, or other convenient foods in your desk drawer. Meal delays happen, wherever you are, so always carry a snack or two in your purse or pocket, and monitor your blood sugar level as needed.

Alcohol:

When the gang invites you to a bar after work, enjoy yourself. But take care regarding the alcohol that you drink:

"Alcohol has two separate problems related to diabetes," says Dr. Stuart Brink, Senior Endocrinologist at the New England Diabetes and Endocrine Center.

One has to do with what type of alcohol you're drinking, because some alcohol will have some sugar effects—beer, if you have a mixed drink, or what you're mixing with orange juice or cola or whatever. It's very straightforward in that aspect, because . . . simple sugars raise your blood sugars rather quickly and sometimes very, very high. So, you need to learn what happens under those circumstances for *you* . . .

A second, more devastating and serious problem with alcohol is that, hours later, alcohol doesn't cause low blood sugars, but makes anything that causes low blood sugar into a potential disaster. And that happens very specifically because alcohol is metabolized, is broken up, is used by the body, through the liver. And when the liver gets busy taking care of alcohol, it . . . doesn't have enough time to take care of your sugar needs. So if you were hypoglycemic at four AM after you have been out dancing, burning up sugars, and drinking—a lot of alcohol in your system blocking your liver now from fixing a low blood sugar—what might be a very mild hypoglycemic reaction, could be an unconscious reaction or a convulsion four, six, ten AM the next morning.

Now, [these effects] don't happen exactly at the same time. The high-sugar part is the first few hours after drinking, and that's the simple sugar effect; and the alcohol effect by itself is four hours, six hours, twelve hours later. But you have to know both of those things.

Having diabetes does not mean that you must avoid alcohol,

but don't go over your personal limit. If you indulge, eat something with your drink to reduce the glucose-lowering effect of the alcohol. Be sure to have a designated driver in your group, and tell at least one of your companions that you have diabetes. If you have a serious problem with alcohol, including alcoholic beverages in your meal plan is not for you.

Party Safely

Always wear medical identification, in case of an emergency. Gone are the days of unattractive-looking metal chain bracelets. Today, you can purchase medical alert bracelets and necklaces that are made with precious and semiprecious stones, charms, modern metallic designs, and even Velcro fastenings. For a great selection, visit childrenwithdiabetes.com and run a search for medical identification.

If an outing with your business associates causes you to miss your regular dinner time, grab a snack from your pocket and continue having fun. Remember to check your blood glucose level from time to time if you are not eating at your regular hour and/or consuming food or drink you do not customarily have at that time of day.

WITH YOUR FAMILY

My in-laws came for dinner and brought desserts... you know, the fattening, traditional ones that some of us just can't have. Then one of them repeated over and over, "Oh, come on, just a little won't hurt you!" Finally, I had to be a bit firm and tell them, "No, I can't and you're really not making this easy for me." To be honest, I'm still not pleased with them for that.

—Heather

Some people have been so hurt by their relatives' lack of sensitivity that the topic is almost too painful to discuss. And some people have very supportive relatives, who occasionally forget about their diabetes:

> I stopped by my parent's home one evening after work and sat in the kitchen to watch Mom busily prepare an elaborate dinner for guests who were arriving shortly. Suddenly, my blood sugar began to drop. I stopped talking and sat motionless. My mother, totally oblivious to my situation, kept on cooking. I began to sweat heavily and became pale, but finally mustered up enough energy to utter, "Sugar!" Mom quickly responded, "I love you too, honey!" I uttered, "Sugar!" a second time, and she answered once again, "I love you too, honey." As the last word left her lips, she suddenly realized what was happening, then overreacted and let out an incredible scream.
> *—Bill*

Supportive family members only need a gentle reminder about your diabetes, but the more challenging ones require special strategies. Let's look at a few of the relatives who are the most difficult:

Dense Darla

No matter how many times you explain your diabetes to her, Darla never understands. You've told her what you prefer to eat, but she doesn't listen. Instead, she continues to prepare her favorite dishes and doesn't give your needs a second thought. Darla doesn't get it and is never going to, so appreciate her for who she is. Find something to talk with her about other than health and food, and accept that she is not going to change. Take the first step to end the vicious circle of trying to make each other feel guilty. Eat before you see her, or bring along something that you can have; if she presses you to sample a food you prefer to avoid, compliment the dish without making any accusations against her—say, "That cake is so beautiful, but I have to say no," or "Oh, that smells so good, but sorry, I've just eaten"—and change the subject immediately to one she loves to discuss.

Pushy Pete

Pete doesn't take your diabetes seriously and believes that you shouldn't, either. He continuously urges you to eat foods that you prefer to avoid and offers you advice that will undermine your goals. Surely you can have a bite of a forbidden food and not tell your doctor, right? When Pete offers his guidance, just listen, smile, and ignore it. You probably aren't going to convince him that you are more knowledgeable than he about what you'd like to consume, are committed to healthy goals, and know what to do to reach them. As with Dense Darla, changing the subject is the way to go, as responding will only increase Pete's desire to win the argument.

Overprotective Olive

Olive views you as a child. She asks everyone to be kind to you because you have a disease. She clips diabetes articles for you whether or not they apply to your particular type of diabetes, repeats dubious advice she has learned from the Internet, is always warning you about possible complications she has heard about, and goes into red alert if you wish to consume what she believes is bad for you. She, of course, has no real understanding of your true condition. It is a challenge to work with Olive, but you can succeed. You have three ways to deal with her:

1. Politely ask her to stop speaking to others on your behalf. Tell her that, while you appreciate her interest in your health, diabetes care has changed over the past few years,

and you and your health-care team know what is best for you.
2. Use her enthusiasm to your advantage. Let her know that your diet has been changed to include particular foods that you enjoy, and ask her to tell everyone about this change. This assignment provides Olive with a helpful task that she will relish. She will also help you spread correct information to the rest of the family.
3. Do exactly what you did with Dense Darla and Pushy Pete—thank her for her concern but then ignore her unsolicited advice, and redirect her zeal to another subject about which she feels she is an expert.

Blaming Bill

Bill resents your diabetes and puts the blame squarely on your shoulders: You allowed yourself to become overweight and ignored your health, so your diabetes is *your* fault. Now, because of your negligence, *he* has to suffer. The whole family is focused on *your* needs, while *his* are totally ignored. Even his favorite fried dishes and gooey desserts are no longer served on holidays, because no one wants to tempt you or throw you off your diet. Well, Bill is totally wrong. Your diabetes is not your fault. Don't let him convince you otherwise. Betty Brackenridge, coauthor of *Diabetes Myths, Misconceptions, and Big Fat Lies*, clarifies this diabetes myth:

> Because people feel guilty, they think somehow they've brought this on themselves. They're less willing to speak up if things aren't going well. They think, "Oh, somehow, it must be my fault." But, it's simply not true. Diabetes is not a character flaw, it's a disease! It's caused by a combination of genetics, so the worst thing you did was to pick your parents. You know, I picked my dad. He had diabetes and, you know, I'll take dad and the diabetes. But the fact I was susceptible to it

was based very much on my genetics, then something in the environment meets up with those genetics and the disease comes out.

In type 1 diabetes, there's a tendency for the immune system to go crazy and beat off the cells in the pancreas that make insulin. In type 2 diabetes, the thing in the environment is really modern life. Those of us who develop type 2 diabetes were survivors [in the days when] people starved a lot and did hard physical work. Now in America, where everybody is getting very little exercise . . . My grandparents who had a ranch and worked the farm would laugh themselves silly that I have to go out and spend money to go to the gym three or four times a week. So, it's not that people are bad, it's that people are living the modern life. We don't want to give up dishwashers and wash dishes by hand again. We don't want to give up washing machines and dryers, and go out and hang up the laundry, or use a push mower on the half acre in the backyard. You know, modern life has created a lot of conveniences and those conveniences have really preyed on people who have this survivor gene.

YOU CAN PICK your friends, but you can't pick your relatives. Fortunately, some relatives will rise to the occasion and offer their support. As for the others who continue to make life difficult for you, just refuse to provide any additional fuel for their negativity, and keep your eye on your goals.

WITH YOUR FRIENDS

BE A WONDERFUL example to those around you by hosting a party that offers healthy fare. Numerous diabetes and heart-smart cookbooks are available, many of which offer simple as well as gourmet recipes. Don't forget to adjust your own favorites by incorporating better ingredients and cooking methods. Here are a few simple choices that you can serve when the guests arrive:

Beverages—Wine mixed with sparkling water; punches made with artificially sweetened sodas; imported spring water in beautiful bottles, served with a twist of lemon or lime; a selection of exotic and herbal teas, or a selection of quality coffees, with optional artificial sweeteners and low-fat milk

Appetizers—Baked chips and salsa; cut raw or blanched vegetables with low-fat or fat-free sour cream–based dips; shrimp and cocktail sauce; hummus and toasted whole wheat pita triangles

Soup—Gazpacho, vegetarian vegetable soup, high-fiber mushroom barley and bean soups

Entrées—Stir-fried vegetables with lean meat, chicken, or tofu; baked chicken (without the skin); lasagne made with a generous amount of vegetables and low-fat cheeses; turkey; lean barbequed meats; vegetable and hummus rolled up in whole-grain tortilla wraps; tuna wraps; homemade pizza with a variety of different toppings on a whole-grain crust, and healthier versions of your favorite dishes

Side dishes—Fresh, steamed, roasted and baked vegetables; salads; a variety of dishes prepared with brown rice and/or other whole grains, beans, nuts, and seeds

Desserts—Low-fat ice cream and frozen yogurts; yogurt parfaits made by layering sugar-free yogurt, low-fat granola, and fresh fruit; baked apples; calorie-free gelatin with low-calorie whipped topping; fresh fruit

Organize a Potluck Party

Invite your friends to a potluck banquet for which *you* supply the recipes. This activity will familiarize them with the foods that you prefer to eat, and introduce them to cooking techniques and ingredients that are good for them as well. If they prefer to choose their own recipes, pass out your favorite diabetes and heart-healthy cookbooks and assign everyone a different course to prepare.

When invited to a party at a friend's house, even if it is not a potluck, offer to bring along a delicious main dish or dessert you know you can eat, to share with the other guests.

FRIENDS WHO TRY to divert you from your dietary goals can be handled in the same way as unhelpful relatives. If your attempts to educate them don't have an impact, enjoy them for who they are, and try to arrange to enjoy their company in situations that do not revolve around food. Look beyond dining for ways to share what has bonded you as friends. Instead of meeting for lunch, for example, spend the day at an event that interests you both, or invite your friends to join you at a restaurant of *your* choosing where you know you can select a healthy meal without fuss.

Out on the Town

> So far, I think the only real noticeable change in my life as a diabetic has been socially. When I'm eating out with a group of friends, sometimes they treat me differently (which I hate). I didn't realize how aggravating it is when a nondiabetic thinks they are trying to help you by chastising your choices in food, when in actuality you are in more control than they can comprehend.
>
> —"Yogiraj"
>
> (from the dearjanis.com message board)

Most people know at least someone who has diabetes. What they don't always know is that treatment and food choices have changed dramatically in recent years, and that you can enjoy snacks and desserts, as long as you select them with care.

Don't shy away from going out with your friends. As mentioned previously, wear medical identification, let at least one of your companions know that you have diabetes, obtain a menu ahead of time if you can, discuss preparation and dressings/sauces with your waitperson, and bring emergency snacks.

Don't assume that food will be available at non-food-related events, such as a theatrical performance or a sporting event. Your group's plans may suddenly change, you may get caught in traffic, or there may be no convenience store nearby. Even if a concessions stand will be available, the chances are good that it will offer fast or prepared foods high in fat, salt, and/or sugar; bring along your own tasty treats whose ingredients you know for sure.

And discomfort can go both ways: don't make your friends feel guilty for ordering foods less healthy than your selections. Their diet is their choice, just as your is yours.

WITH A DATE

DATING IS STRESSFUL, whether you have diabetes or not. You worry about what to say, do, eat, drink, wear, and on and on. If you have diabetes, a date can turn into quite an interesting adventure:

> I dated back in the "dark ages" of diabetes. I did have a home glucose meter—the big ones you had to plug in for an hour and calibrate (needle display—nothing digital) for high and low before testing with a huge amount of blood and waiting a total of 2 minutes before inserting the strip in the meter. Needless to say, I didn't test often or carry the meter around. I was starting to get serious with my now husband of 25 years,

and we went to church together on a beautiful spring day. I'd spoken with him a little about diabetes and hypoglycemia, but hadn't made a big deal out of it. It was about a 1.5 mile walk to and from church. On the way home I became hypoglycemic and started acting very drunk. We are members of the Church of Jesus Christ of Latter-Day Saints, better known as the Mormon Church, so we do not consume alcohol! Anyway, he remained very calm and attentive and when a car stopped to ask if we need help, he got both of us into it, took me into my second-story apartment, and poured me some juice. Needless to say, he was a keeper! After being initially embarrassed, I decided it was a good experience because it evaluated his ability to deal with the worst of my condition.
—Eileen

Fortunately, for a person with diabetes, even dating has changed. What hasn't changed, however, is the fact that at some point in your relationship, you must disclose that you have diabetes. Different people handle this in different ways.

Some people make an official announcement and others let their diabetes speak for itself—they do their diabetes-care tasks openly and answer any questions that arise. The more relaxed you are about your diabetes, the more relaxed your date will be. If you give the impression that your diabetes is a terrible inconvenience or embarrassment, he or she will believe that as well. Do what is comfortable for you, but make sure that you don't neglect your diabetes during your date. Your health is too important.

If your date seems squeamish, ask the person a few questions to determine whether he or she has any misconceptions about diabetes. You may need to offer reassurance that you are not ill, or that the testing and injections do not hurt, or that with treatment you may never develop the diabetes complications he/she may have heard about. (Think back to when you were first diagnosed: you probably found it scary and confusing, too, because you didn't know much about it.) Stress that you are healthy and that, by taking care of yourself, you are living a full life. But if, despite your best efforts to put your date at ease, the person gives off negative vibes about your being diabetic, remember: there is nothing about this condition that you should feel apologetic or secretive about. If he/she is not understanding, you may have to decide whether it is really worthwhile for you to become involved with someone so unsupportive of your needs. The upside is that there are plenty of potential partners as empathetic as Eileen's.

STEP 14

Prepare for Intimacy

IF YOU EXPECT to become physical with your significant other, check your blood glucose frequently and treat hypoglycemic symptoms with glucose tablets or a fast-acting carbohydrate food, such as regular soda or fruit juice. Sex is a physical activity just like running and dancing, and can cause your blood sugar level to drop quickly.

As mentioned earlier, diabetes can affect sexual performance. Men may have a difficult time achieving or maintaining an erection or may experience a drop in libido; and women may have difficulty becoming aroused, may lack adequate vaginal lubrication, have difficulty achieving orgasm, or feel pain during intercourse. There are many treatments available. If your first choice doesn't work out, try another. Don't let diabetes rob you of one of the most important connections that you can have with a loved one.

MEN'S DIABETES-RELATED SEXUAL ISSUES

HERE ARE SOME of these treatments for erectile dysfunction (ED):

- *Improved blood sugar control*—This will help prevent problems from occurring and can improve them once they develop.
- *Blood pressure control*—You need to keep the blood vessels in this region of the body as healthy as possible. If your blood pressure is not at a normal level, it may be more difficult for you to achieve and maintain an erection.
- *Blood lipid (fats) and cholesterol control*—It helps to keep blood vessels clear, so adequate blood flow can reach the penis.
- *Regular physical activity*—Exercise helps improve circulation, reduces blood pressure, increases energy, improves the body's sensitivity to insulin, heightens feelings of well being, and improves blood sugar control.
- *Counseling, with or without a partner*—Some cases of ED occur because of emotional problems or stress. If you aren't attracted to your partner, are angry, or feel dissatisfied with the relationship, counseling may help put things back into a healthy perspective.
- *Vacuum pumps, constriction rings, and penile support sleeves*—These tools work, but you must learn to use them properly. If you have any questions about how to use one of these items, ask your health-care provider to refer you to someone who can teach you the correct way to use it.
- *Oral agents, such as Viagra, Levitra, and Cialis*—These pills are frequently offered as a first option. They work for many men, but not all. If you don't get the results that you expect, contact your physician.
- *Penile suppositories and injections*—Many men find these extremely helpful. The injections may sound gruesome, but they work quite well.
- *Surgical treatments, such as semi-rigid and inflatable penile implants*—These work also, but must be surgically implanted and should only be considered after all other options have failed.

WOMEN'S DIABETES-RELATED SEXUAL ISSUES

FEW WOMEN REALIZE that diabetes can affect their ability to have a meaningful sexual experience. Poor diabetes control can cause mood swings, decreased interest in being sexual, vaginal dryness, decreased sensitivity, problems with achieving orgasm, and yeast and urinary tract infections. Many of the women's treatments for diabetes–related sexual issues are similar to the men's. They include:

- Improved blood sugar control
- Blood pressure control
- Blood lipid (fats) and cholesterol control
- Physical activity, which improves circulation, reduces blood pressure, helps increase energy, improves the body's sensitivity to insulin, heightens feelings of well being, and can help improve blood sugar control
- Counseling, with or without a partner
- Vaginal lubricants, such as K-Y, Replens, and Astroglide to help increase vaginal lubrication and reduce pain during intercourse
- Vibrating tools to help encourage lubrication and orgasm. This can help if you have reduced sensitivity in the vaginal area
- Masturbation to help encourage lubrication and orgasm
- Counseling to help learn ways to achieve orgasm and handle feelings of depression and loss of self-esteem

If you have a urinary or vaginal infection, it can interfere with your intimate life also. Diabetes can cause them to develop, and abnormal blood sugar levels will make them occur more frequently. Symptoms of a yeast infection include vaginal itching, irritated skin in the genital area, pain while urinating, burning or pain in the genital area during intercourse, and an odorless, white vaginal discharge that resembles cottage cheese. Symptoms of a urinary tract infection include pain or burning when you urinate, a frequent urge to urinate small amounts, cloudy or foul-smelling urine, pain on the side of your back under your ribcage, fever, chills, nausea, vomiting, and a feeling of tenderness in your lower abdomen.

Speak with your physician or gynecologist if you have any of the symptoms listed above. There are several over-the-counter medications that you can use to treat vaginal infections, but you should first confirm that this is what you have. To help prevent these conditions from developing, keep your blood sugar level in a normal range, wear cotton underwear, eat low-fat yogurt that contains active cultures, drink plenty of water, drink artificially sweetened cranberry juice, bathe regularly, wipe the genital area from front to back after going to the bathroom (to avoid introducing new bacteria into the vaginal area), and only participate in intimate activities with a partner who has recently bathed.

MOST PEOPLE ARE uncomfortable discussing intimate issues. If you feel that way, you are not alone. Don't let your discomfort prevent you from receiving help. Speak with a health-care provider whom you trust and believe will be sensitive to your needs, and discuss with your partner what might enhance your experience together.

CHOOSE YOUR JUMP-START PLEDGE

- I pledge to carry my glucose meter wherever I go this week.
- I pledge to carry several healthy snacks whenever I go out this week.
- I pledge to say yes this week to a social invitation I have been avoiding because of dining issues.

- I plan to handle differently this week one relative or friend's comments about my food choices.
- I pledge to check my glucose level before intimate activity this week.
- I pledge to wear medical identification for one week.
- I pledge to [your choice] for one week.

TAKE CHARGE

Enjoy a healthy and vigorous social life . . . on your own terms!

8

SAY YES TO . . .
A Less Stressful Life

MANY OF MY patients are surprised when I inquire about the physical and emotional stress in their lives. Most don't realize the affect that this can have on their diabetes control, overall feeling of well being, health, and ability to take care of their diabetes. No one's life is without stress. Fortunately, there are several actions that you can take to reduce the intensity of your world. Let's review them:

IN THIS CHAPTER, YOU WILL:

- Learn the effects of stress on your physical health.
- Explore ways to reduce the level of stress in your life.
- Reorganize your Jump-Start Pledges to help reduce stress.
- Make another Jump-Start Pledge.

STEP 15

Reduce the Stress in Your Life

A RABBI ONCE GAVE A FRIEND THE FOLLOWING BLESSING: "I PRAY THAT YOUR LIFE BE FILLED WITH MANY SMALL PROBLEMS." THE FRIEND WAS SHOCKED. WHAT KIND OF BLESSING IS THAT? THE RABBI EXPLAINED, "WHEN YOU HAVE MANY SMALL PROBLEMS IN YOUR LIFE, YOU DON'T HAVE ANY LARGE ONES. IF SOMEONE IS SERIOUSLY ILL, DO YOU CARE IF YOUR DRY CLEANING IS NOT DONE ON TIME? DO CARE IF YOU BRING HOME THE WRONG BRAND OF SALAD DRESSING? NO. YOU ARE SO FOCUSED ON YOUR LOVED ONE'S ILLNESS THAT YOU DON'T NOTICE THE SMALL ANNOYANCES THAT OCCUR EACH DAY. THAT IS WHY I OFFER YOU THIS BLESSING. MAY YOUR LIFE BE FILLED WITH SMALL PROBLEMS, FOR IF IT IS, YOU HAVE NO MAJOR ONES TO WORRY ABOUT."
—*adapted from a story by Rabbi Abraham J. Twerski, MD*

•

PHYSICAL STRESS FROM a cold, infection, or illness can raise your blood glucose level and make it harder to control. When you are overscheduled and are pulled in numerous directions, your time ceases to be your own. Is it possible that you are stressed and don't know it? Sure. We have an amazing ability to accommodate ourselves to our environment. Many of us don't truly appreciate how hectic our lives are. We don't realize the level of stress that we live with each day until something extreme happens—either we go on vacation and the tension comes noticeably to a halt, or we are hit with an even more challenging responsibility that we feel we cannot handle on top of the rest, or we become ill.

When people are stressed, their health will suffer. They may have difficulty falling asleep, gain weight, drink too much caffeine or alcohol, develop high blood pressure, or experience mood swings. If you have diabetes, you may experience additional issues: Your blood sugar level can be more difficult to control and you may ignore important self-care tasks, such as daily foot inspections, regular physical activity, and blood tests. You may even forget to take your medication.

When your tension level drops, on the other hand, you can think more clearly, feel more energetic, and even sleep better. Your body will also break down carbohydrates more efficiently, which helps normalize your blood glucose level.

Here are several ways to help you reduce the stress in your life and take charge once again:

Have Realistic Expectations

In the first chapter, we discussed how important it is to realize that perfect diabetes control is not possible. If you try to be perfect all of the time, you will probably become very distraught. You may also become upset when your health-care providers don't perform as you expect them to, especially if you and your doctor don't see eye-to-eye when it comes to your diabetes care. Sometimes you must be assertive to make that happen, says Betty Brackenridge, coauthor of *Diabetes Myths, Misconceptions, and Big Fat Lies*:

> One of the biggest problems is that a lot of providers assume that people know certain things about their diabetes and would or wouldn't be willing to do certain kinds of therapy. They try to make things easy on people instead of helping them be the best they can be. So, if a person with diabetes has great information and knows what they want, they can go to their doctor and say, "Hey, don't leave this exam room yet. You're supposed to check my feet every time I'm in here." Or, "Why haven't you mentioned a new pill or new insulin that's available. It sounds to me like it might be helpful."

It is important to recognize the role that each member of your health-care team plays in your overall well-being. If you consult a health-care professional who is also a certified diabetes educator (CDE), you should be able to get answers to diabetes-related questions, regardless of the topic. But providers who are not CDEs may not be able to adequately respond to questions outside their area of specialization:

> I called my new registered dietitian to ask her a question about my insulin dose. She told me to call my endo. I got so angry. Why couldn't she answer my question? Doesn't she know anything?
> —Paula

If Paula, a regular visitor to the dearjanis.com message board, had asked her a question about nutrition, meal planning, or weight loss, she would have received a helpful response. Not all registered dietitians, however, know detailed information about insulin use. For that, Paula needed to consult a dietitian who is also a CDE. When the dietitian told Paula to contact her endocrinologist, she wasn't ignoring her inquiry; she was providing her with a way to get a quality response. It can be frustrating to expect help from someone who doesn't know an answer, but before you get too aggravated, be sure that you have asked the appropriate individual your question.

Revise Your Schedule

J. Anthony Brown, a comedian, host of *dLifeTV*, and radio personality who lives in Los Angeles, has a challenging schedule. Each morning, he wakes up at two AM (Pacific time) to cohost the *Tom Joyner Morning Show*, which broadcasts simultaneously from several locations in the United States. When the show ends at seven AM, J. Anthony returns to bed. This schedule is not only grueling, it affects his diabetes control, eating patterns, and exercise schedule. J. Anthony recently decided to put his health first and move to a more convenient time zone than the one he lived in on the West Coast:

> I've been in LA for about fourteen or fifteen years. I've made a lot of friends, I have a home out there, my dogs out there, my business is out there, but for health reasons, if I was [starting the show in New York at] 11 o'clock at night, I could go to bed and still get a nice rest, as opposed to trying to jump up at two o'clock in the morning and do a radio show . . . I want to live a healthy life and I want to enjoy some of the fruits of my labor.

J. Anthony's situation is an extreme one. You probably don't have to move to reduce your stress level, but you may have to make some serious changes. Review your current schedule and see what you can do to make your day less hectic. If necessary, resign from volunteer committees, stop associating with people who bother you, take time for lunch each day, and, if you work at home, set a specific time to end your work for the evening.

Don't Burn the Midnight Oil

Do you get the sleep that you need? According to the National Sleep Foundation, many of us sleep poorly, which affects our professional relationships, productivity, public safety, and even our personal lives.

- Nearly one fourth of adults in relationships have infrequent sex because they are too sleepy.
- Sixty percent of adults say that they have driven while too tired.

- Four percent have had an accident or near accident because of fatigue or have dozed off at the wheel.

If you are tired a nap could be helpful, but don't rest longer than twenty to forty minutes, or it will be more difficult to sleep later that evening. Avoid eating or drinking too much before bedtime, and complete any physical activity at least three hours before you turn in for the night. Avoid caffeine, nicotine, and alcohol later in the day. Caffeine and nicotine can make it more difficult to fall asleep and alcohol may interfere with your sleep later in the night. Upsetting news can also keep you awake, so turn off the television, computer, or other attention-commanding electronic media at least one hour prior to bedtime.

Wind down as bedtime nears. Listen to soothing music, soak in a warm bath, or read. Try to make your bedroom as inviting as possible: cool, comfortable, quiet, and dark. Use it exclusively for sleeping, so that you will be primed for sleep whenever you are there. If you don't fall asleep within fifteen minutes, leave the bedroom and do a relaxing activity such as reading, then return when you feel fatigued.

When should you go to bed? Elizabeth Trattner, a nationally recognized acupuncture physician, encourages her patients to be in bed before eleven PM. She says that, according to Chinese medicine's understanding of how we function, our body begins to recharge its internal battery at that hour. Don't miss out on this important opportunity to rejuvenate yourself. Do your best to get under the sheets at a reasonable time. If sleep is a problem for you, seek professional help.

Stay Active

Physical activity is a terrific way to improve your health and relieve stress. Be sure to include some form of activity in your day. See chapter 2 for more discussion of this.

Enjoy Water Therapy

There is nothing like a soothing bath to end a hectic day. Individuals with diabetes are often cautioned against bathing for extended periods of time because it can cause the skin to dry out and crack, which increases the risk of infection. But as long as you exit the water before the pads of your fingers and toes "prune" or shrivel, you should be fine. If you have lost some sensitivity in your feet, check the temperature of the water before stepping in. This warning goes for hot tubs as well. The water in a hot tub is extremely hot and can cause a serious burn if you have diabetic neuropathy and are unable to feel the heat with your feet or legs. Hot tub use may help reduce blood glucose levels in some people with type 2 diabetes but, if you have heart disease, you should limit your time in the tub to less than twenty or thirty minutes, or your blood pressure might drop.

When you bathe, try aromatherapy, a treatment that employs high-quality plant-derived essential oils to help promote a feeling of well-being. Fragrant oils have been enjoyed throughout history, as far back as the time of the ancient Greeks and Romans. These scents can calm, improve alertness, increase relaxation, and even heighten sexual interest. Essential oils can be rubbed into the skin during massage therapy, warmed so they distribute into the air, or added to bath water. They are available at most health food stores.

Those known to help relieve stress include:

- Lavender
- Chamomile
- Geranium
- Sandalwood
- Juniper berry
- Sweet marjoram

Relax Your Mind, Body, and Soul

A Korean study observed the effect that soothing music had on patients admitted to a hospital with a heart attack. Those who heard the music showed fewer signs of stress than did the individuals who did not receive musical treatment. In Sweden, a group of patients were operated on as music played. After surgery, they had less pain and anxiety than individuals who were operated on in silence. In another study done at the University of Kansas, researchers found that music decreased the anxiety and sleep patterns of abused women in shelters. Listen to soothing music when you feel stressed. It may help you as well.

Massage helps relieve muscle tension that lingers from a stressful moment or event. When you encounter a stress-filled situation, your muscles tense up, heart rate and blood pressure increase, breathing may quicken, and hormones adrenaline and norepinephrine get released. A massage helps return your body to a calmer state. It also improves circulation, relieves pain, promotes healing, and helps you sleep better. Massage offers benefits for diabetes control as well. It may increase insulin absorption at injection sites, improve blood glucose levels, and relieve symptoms of diabetic neuropathy. Massage can also help relieve a variety of physical injuries from overexerting during exercise, wearing the wrong shoes, sitting at a computer for too long, carrying heavy packages, or participating in other challenges to your body and posture. Numerous types of massage range from the oiled rubbing of a Swedish massage to the sharp pressing of shiatsu.

Yoga, when done correctly, can help improve blood glucose control, increase flexibility, and promote relaxation. The gentle stretching relieves tension throughout the body, and the deep, rhythmic breathing encourages a soothing and meditative response. Numerous styles of yoga include the gentle stretching of Iyengar, the meditative style of Kripalu, and the intensely aerobic and fast-paced Ashtanga. If you wish to study yoga, discuss your physical needs and goals with the staff of a certified yoga center. Certain styles will be more appropriate for you than others.

Meditation can improve your overall health, lift your spirit, and relax you. Nina Yarus, a meditation teacher in Miami, supports meditation as a tool for stress-reduction and even, in some instances, medication reduction:

> The incredible thing about meditation is that no matter what physical shape you're in, no matter where you are geographically, or even if you don't have time, you can do meditation. Five minutes is better than no minutes and you will absolutely see an impact when you begin to meditate.

Ten to twenty minutes of meditation each day reduces blood pressure, relieves muscle tension, and improves your heart rate. Studies have shown that it helps fight off illness and infection, and may enhance your attention, memory, and learning. There are many ways to meditate. Here is one way that Nina recommends that you begin:

1. Sit up in bed with your spine erect. Your legs can be in any position that is comfortable for you.
2. Repeat a phrase of some sort that is positive and soothing. It can be a word, a short line that moves you, a prayer, or even a song.
3. Keep repeating your phrase over and over again. Eventually your breathing will become very quiet.
4. If your mind wanders, just acknowledge that you are thinking of something other than your chosen phrase and begin repeating your phrase once again.

There are many other ways to enjoy the experience of meditation in your life. Find someone who can teach you, read a book on the topic, or listen to an instructional tape. Meditation offers an easy and healthy way to relieve a lot of stress.

Tap into the Power of Prayer

Connecting spiritually to a higher power can help reduce your stress as well. It can bring emotional relief and soothe a troubled mind. But the benefits go beyond the emotions. Researchers at the Medical University of South Carolina found that people with diabetes who regularly attend religious services had lower levels of an inflammatory risk factor for cardiovascular disease known as C-reactive protein, than did those who didn't attend services. Being part of a supportive and welcoming community may be part of the reason for this benefit as it can help reduce a person's stress level. Certain religious practices are also beneficial—they encourage a calmer lifestyle and may discourage use of alcohol, nicotine, and caffeine. Orthodox Jews observe a complete day of rest each week during which no work-related tasks, such as talking on the phone, writing, or using the computer, are permitted. This offers members of that group a very intense release from the pressures of the week. Whatever type of spiritual connection you have, enjoy the health benefits that it brings to your life.

Reevaluate Your Use of Jump-Start Pledges

Throughout this book, I've suggested numerous Jump-Start Pledges for you to try. When you begin new health-related behaviors in small, easy doses, you should feel less overwhelmed by the changes, because you are controlling what they are and how they are fitting into your overall lifestyle. If you've already attempted to do some of these, great! Here are some thoughts from folks from the dearjanis.com message board, who have successfully used this technique:

> I'm going to renew my pledge to do at least 2,500 steps at least 4 days this week, and 3,000 steps for 2 days. I did well at it this past week,

hitting my target 6 out of 7 days. So this week bumps it up two days per week from that level.
—Mary

•

My pledge this week: not eating after 8 PM. Works for me! Jump-Start Pledges have really changed my diabetic life. I would not be reaching my goals without the JSP.
—"Red"

•

I like the Jump-Start Pledge. It has given me something to strive for. It makes me commit to a goal and be accountable. It has created good habits and made me let go of bad ones. It has been said "It takes 21 days to develop a habit." I firmly believe this. In my Jump-Start pledge I pledged to exercise for the majority of the week. I have met that goal and now it's a habit.
—"Clee"

•

I do like the idea of little steps at a time. It definitely makes each change easier to do. Nothing seems too big. This week I am trying to get to bed by 9:30.
—Sharon

•

Everyone began with a single pledge. After several weeks of renewing that pledge, many were ready to add another and possibly a third. They were not trying to make every possible change all at once.

Sundar (Sunny) lives in Bangalore, India, is an active participant on the dearjanis.com board, and is a fan of Jump-Start Pledges. They work so well for him, that he created a special form to help keep track of them. As you can see, Sunny has listed several Jump-Start Pledges, but he initially began with a single goal.

PLEDGE FOR WEEK 1

WEEK 1

PLEDGE	MON	TUE	WED	THR	FRI	SAT	SUN
Should get to bed before 11:00							
Drink water throughout the day							
Avoid eating after 8:30 PM							
Spend at least 30 minutes on physical work							
Follow up and get pedometer							
Check BS every morning							

Diabetes self-care tasks can seem quite daunting. Don't let them overwhelm you. You can use something like Sunny's chart, and check off your pledges each day that you successfully complete them. Don't choose more than one pledge at first. When you feel ready, add another until you have several. Think about which new pledges you would like to try, incorporate them into your life one by one as you become comfortable with those you have already made, and in time you should see some very impressive results.

Kiss Your Partner . . . and Fido

Your partner may seem to be a source of tension but, according to researchers at the University of Toronto, an attentive and sympathetic partner can reduce your blood pressure and help combat the effects of a stressful job. Another loved one who is always willing to hear you gripe about your day is a loving pet. A dog or cat can significantly lower your heart rate and calm you during a stressful time. Elderly individuals who have pets visit their doctor less frequently, and AIDS patients who have pets have a lower incidence of depression. So appreciate your partner—and your loving Rover and Fluffy—each evening when you return home from work.

STEP 16

Seek Help For Depression, If Needed

A DISCUSSION OF stress is not complete without mentioning the topic of depression. Throughout this book, I have emphasized the value of making your own decisions and choosing your own diabetes destiny. If you are depressed, you will have difficulty doing that. You may be overwhelmed by feelings that you can't shake off and don't understand. If you have diabetes, your risk for developing depression actually doubles: approximately 30 percent of individuals who have diabetes also experience depression. It doesn't make a difference if you have type 1 or type 2, the rates of depression in both groups is about the same. We do know, however, that depression is more common in women than men and that it tends to increase when diabetes complications become present. You should seek help for this, if this applies to you. You deserve to live the life that you have always wanted, and shouldn't permit feelings of depression to stop you from this worthwhile goal.

We don't fully understand the relationship between diabetes and depression. Here is a list of recognized symptoms of major depression that were highlighted in *Newsflash*, a publication of the Diabetes Care and Education, a Dietetic Practice Group of the American Dietetic Association:

- Depressed mood (feeling sad, "blue," cheerless)
- Loss of interest in things usually enjoyed
- Feelings of guilt or worthlessness
- Persistent anxiety, worry, or "empty" mood
- Increased/decreased appetite
- Decreased energy level
- Decreased ability to concentrate, make decisions
- Difficulty remembering things
- Sleeping too much/too little
- Feeling restless/irritable
- Thought of death or suicide
- Loss of self-esteem
- Withdrawal from friends/family
- Increased crying
- Substance abuse
- Persistent physical pains that don't go away

Only 75 percent of people with diabetes seek help for their depression symptoms. If you experience any symptoms that you believe may be signs of depression and they don't improve within a reasonable period of time, upset you, or begin to interfere with your daily life, speak with a member of your health-care team.

CHOOSE YOUR JUMP-START PLEDGE

- I pledge to take a relaxing bath every evening for a week.
- I pledge to do some form of stretching or yoga for at least 10 minutes each day this week.
- I pledge to meditate for 10 minutes each day this week.
- I plan to add 30 minutes of "quality time" with my pet every evening for a week.
- I pledge to turn off my [television, video/DVD player/computer] at least an hour before bedtime every day this week.
- I plan to go to bed an hour earlier every day this week.
- I pledge to [your choice] for one week.

TAKE CHARGE

RELIEVE YOUR STRESS AND DEPRESSION, TO BE THE BEST YOU CAN BE.

9

SAY YES TO...
Roads Well (and Less) Traveled

SHARI, A PATIENT of mine, was a wreck. Her husband had recently retired and wanted to see the world, but she was afraid to join him. She recently developed type 2 diabetes and was just starting to feel comfortable with all of the changes that came with it. The thought of strange food, time changes, and an unpredictable day was frightening. "How do people with diabetes travel?"

IN THIS CHAPTER, YOU WILL:

- Overcome your fear of traveling with diabetes.
- Read the story of the first solo flight around the world by a pilot with diabetes.
- Learn how to travel successfully and safely with diabetes.
- Develop a packing list for different modes of travel.
- Review domestic and international travel issues.
- Make a new Jump-Start Pledge.

STEP 17

Don't Let Diabetes Stop You

DON'T LET DIABETES keep you from exploring different cultures, visiting famous locales, and tasting new cuisine. If you haven't traveled a lot or feel nervous about heading far from home, a trip may seem overwhelming. Schedule a practice run at a nearby hotel. You will be away for a night or two, yet be close to home in case of an emergency. Here is how Dave, one of my patients, faced his travel concerns:

> DAVE *has type 2 diabetes. He and his wife Nancy wanted to head out west, but worried about Dave's diabetes needs. They haven't enjoyed a real vacation since Dave was diagnosed about four years ago. After having a blood sugar low while driving to visit some relatives, they began to shy away from out-of-town family gatherings. This, of course, brought a level of stress into the marriage. They both wanted to go out, but Dave felt that he needed to stay home. Diabetes was robbing them of an enormous amount of fun. Finally, they decided to turn things around. They booked a weekend at a nearby hotel to see if they could successfully spend the night away. This small trip would be their trial run.*
>
> *First, they created a checklist of things that Dave might need. It included extra diabetes supplies and workout clothes to wear in the hotel's exercise facility. Initially he felt nervous about sleeping in an unfamiliar bed, so he packed his pillow, which helped him fall right to sleep. By the time they returned home, they felt ready to travel for a slightly longer trip, a bit farther away from home. They hope to book a trip to the Grand Canyon sometime next year.*

Once you get more comfortable, you should be able to go anywhere with confidence . . . even around the world.

When Douglas Cairns, a flight instructor with Britain's Royal Air Force, was diagnosed with diabetes, he immediately lost his pilot's license. After several years, he finally regained it and became the first person with type 1 diabetes to fly solo around the world. Here is an excerpt from a discussion that I had with him on my radio show:

> When I was flying jets in the Royal Air Force at the age of twenty-five, I basically came down with all the classic symptoms of type 1 diabetes. And when I went to the doctor, he took a urine test and turned around to me and said, "You are a diabetic and you were a pilot." Well, I was devastated . . . having to face up to the fact that I wouldn't be able to fly anymore . . . it was a bitter blow to have to take . . . For the first two years, I found it very difficult to adjust. I went from flying my Jet Provost TMark5 to having to work for a living and fly a "mahogany desk Mark 2." Yes, it was really tough to adapt to having one's wings clipped, well and truly.
>
> Occasionally, I would go to flying clubs, and I would grab an instructor who would act as a safety pilot and I would go flying. And basically, I didn't do it enough to be really proficient in the first few years; it was just really to dust a few cobwebs away and have some fun. But I did find that it was a bit of a bittersweet experience, because I loved the flying and it was great to be able to do that. But of course, when I got back on the ground, I'd think, well, it's a damn shame I still can't do that professionally.
>
> It all came about in 1999 when I discovered to my great delight that, here in the USA, a system had been recently introduced that could allow someone with insulin-dependent diabetes to fly on a full, unrestricted private pilot's license. And when I heard about it, I just jumped. In 2000, I was just overjoyed to meet the medical requirements . . . That really sparked another dream that I'd had for really quite some time. I'd always been fascinated by 'round-the-world flights in tiny aircraft . . . And when I realized I possibly could get a license back, I suddenly thought, "You know, why don't you do a world flight of your own, and use it to raise awareness of diabetes and also raise funds for diabetes research?"

And he did. Douglas' flight took 159 days and was made up of multiple stops in different countries. To learn more about his amazing flight, read *Dare to Dream—Flying Solo with Diabetes*.

Whether you are on a brief road trip or off to a distant land, you should:

- *Pack extra food and emergency snacks*—Most travelers run into delays—traffic jams, long lines at check-in counters and security checkpoints, missed connections, lost tickets, even weather delays. Don't assume that an open store or fully stocked snack bar will always be nearby. Always carry food that doesn't require refrigeration, such as diabetes meal replacement drinks, granola bars, fruit, and peanut butter crackers. Carry glucose tablets or other portable, fast-acting carbohydrates to treat unexpected blood sugar lows, and keep water handy to drink if your high blood glucose level starts to run high.
- *Bring diabetes supplies*—Take a generous amount of diabetes supplies with you, including test strips, lancets, batteries, oral medication, insulin, alcohol swabs, and syringes or pens. Certain items may not be available at your final destination, especially if you visit a different country. Insulin, for example, sometimes goes by different names and strengths outside of the United States. If you must purchase some while there, check that the type and concentration are comparable to what you use at home. And keep copies of your prescriptions handy in case your supplies become lost, ruined, or stolen. If you are flying, be sure to carry whatever medications you may need for the actual flight, in the original prescription containers; do not transfer them into other, unmarked containers or they may not be permitted on board.

Opened vials of insulin can be kept at room temperature for 28 to 30 days, as long as they are stored away from direct heat and temperatures greater than 86°F. Refrigerated, unopened vials should last until their expiration dates. Cartridges and prefilled pens kept at room temperature generally last for 10 to 28 days, but check your specific brand of insulin for details. If you are in an extremely hot climate you will need to keep your insulin cool. Be wary of small hotel room refrigerators, as they have erratic temperature controls that may freeze your insulin and destroy its effectiveness, or may not be cool enough to be effective. Instead, purchase a specially made travel pack that offers temperature protection. A home cooler can be used, but don't allow your insulin vial to touch the ice.

- *Take along a first aid kit*—Pick up a small first aid kit at a local pharmacy and add anything that you feel is missing. It should include antibiotic cream, alcohol swabs, bandages, diarrhea and headache medication, bug repellent, sunscreen, and hand and foot cream to maintain your skin while away.
- *Medical identification*—Always wear a medical bracelet, necklace, or other item that identifies you as a person who has diabetes. A card in your wallet or purse can easily become separated from you. In case of an accident or emergency, medical professionals need to know that you require special attention.

STEP 18

Expect the Unexpected

ALEIA *is a professional dancer with type 1 diabetes, who performs all over the world. She has traveled through and lived in Switzerland, Greece, Tahiti, South Africa, French Polynesia, and several countries in the Middle East and Europe. A seasoned traveler, even she has had a glitch or two:*

"Once, while camping in Greece, my insulin went bad because a fellow camper left it out in the sun. I had to search for medical help in a tiny village out in the middle of nowhere. The doctor, who was freshly out of medical school told me, 'I can't help. I don't know anything about diabetes, so get back to Athens as fast as you can.' But I never let these setbacks get me down." Aleia made it safely to Athens and continued on her way.

WHILE TRAVELING, MONITOR your blood glucose level often. You may feel fine, but the stress of adjusting to a new time zone, or just having having a new sleep schedule, varied eating habits, different medication times, and a changed physical activity routine can affect your blood glucose control. You will probably walk more as you explore your new surroundings, its museums, and sights. You may also become so engrossed in a tour that you don't notice low blood glucose symptoms that would normally catch your attention, or symptoms may appear more quickly as your physical activity increases. Insulin is often absorbed more quickly in warmer climates, so be prepared for possible blood sugar lows. If you plan to travel internationally, it may be helpful to learn a few medically related words in the language of that country to help you in an emergency situation.

Test frequently, but don't be disappointed if your normally tight control is a bit off. A vacation is an ideal time to relax your control slightly as long as you remain within a healthy target range. If you travel to a different time zone, discuss with your health-care team any adjustments that you may have to make in your medication schedule. If you head east, your travel day will be shorter, so you may require less insulin. If you head west, you may need additional insulin.

PREPARE FOR YOUR SPECIFIC MODE OF TRAVEL

If You Fly

Food is no longer served on every flight, so bring a generous supply of snacks; you may experience a delay and need something to eat. If food is being served, you can order a low-carbohydrate diabetes meal at least 24 hours ahead of time; as you board, be sure to ask an attendant to confirm that the meal has been loaded onto your flight. Individual airline Web sites provide information about the foods they serve. Here is a sample of a typical airline's diabetic fare:

> *Coach-class Breakfast*—Plain bagel, unsalted margarine, low-calorie jelly and fruit. Meal may also include scrambled eggs, turkey, and Canadian ham

> *Coach-class Lunch*—Smoked turkey sandwich with apple

> *Coach-class Dinner*—Chicken entrée, roll and unsalted margarine. May include salad with dressing and fruit appetizer

Most domestic flights no longer provide meals, but sell snacks. Unfortunately, these convenience store–type snacks tend to be high in salt, sugar, and fat. Your best bet is to pack your own food or purchase a meal at an airport eatery and bring it with you on the plane, if that is permitted.

Take care when packing your items. Place your medications and diabetes-related items in your carry-on bag. Checked bags can become lost and may be subjected to temperature and pressure extremes that can harm your insulin or alter the functioning of your insulin pens. If you have medication that requires refrigeration, purchase a carrying case that keeps it cool. Flight attendants are not usually able to provide refrigeration.

Before entering the security area, tell the screener that you have diabetes and are carrying medical supplies. The FAA recommends that your supplies be clearly labeled and that you carry copies of prescriptions that state the item's name and physician's contact information. Insulin can withstand a brief trip through the security x-ray without any damage. If, however, it remains in the machine for a while or is subjected to multiple x-ray examinations, it could damage its stability. You can always request a personal inspection if you wish to avoid any problems. Keep your supplies in a separate travel pack to expedite this procedure. Inspect your insulin before you take each dose. If you notice anything unusual about its appearance, don't use it and contact a pharmacist or your physician for further instructions.

If you wear an insulin pump, bring a doctor's note that states this fact. You should be able to walk through the security area without any problem. If you are questioned, it is appropriate to let the screener know that your pump cannot be removed because it is attached to your body.

Be patient and informative if you encounter a screener who is unfamiliar with your devices, or who may need to perform extra security measures due to greater circumstances that have made the airport screening unusually arduous.

> JOHN, *a longtime friend of mine, runs a company that imports a variety of products from China. In his capacity as the president/CEO, he travels extensively with several of his business associates. His early visits to China were a bit challenging for a variety of reasons. He had to get used to the time change, the food, the lack of diet Coke (!), and the fact that some of the security inspectors in the smaller airports were not familiar with his insulin pump.*
>
> *On one of his trips, John landed in a smaller city and headed directly to the security check area. As requested, he stood on a box and put his arms out, which permitted the guard to wand him with a handheld metal detector. Each time the wand passed over his pump, it beeped. The guard became*

suspicious and demanded a closer look. John lifted his shirt to show the pump and the infusion set (tubing) that runs from the pump to an adhesive patch on his abdomen. The guard was puzzled. He had never seen a contraption such as this before. "Medicine, medicine," John called out to the guard. An associate who was traveling with John jumped in and added, "Diabetes, diabetes." The guard still didn't know what to make of this item, so he motioned to John to remove it and send it through the x-ray machine. As he disconnected, his friend suggested that John demonstrate the workings of the pump. John set it down and pushed a few buttons to release a few droplets of insulin. Upon seeing the clear liquid come out of the end of the flexible tubing, the guard, and several others who had joined him, broke into huge smiles. They finally understood. The inspection ended on a positive note, with several of the other guards commenting that they had seen many things, but never anything quite like this. John and his co-worker received a voucher for free drinks and all left the area quite pleased. John says, "I travel extensively throughout the United States and China. The folks in security know me by face and refer to me as 'that pump guy.' And every airport security official in China now knows what a pump looks like and what it does. I never have to answer questions anymore."

Once in flight, you may wish to order a beverage. Request the actual beverage can, not just a cup, so that you can identify the source of your drink; don't assume that the flight attendants will bring you the diet item that you've requested. They may become distracted and can easily pour you a nondiet drink. If you order an alcoholic beverage, remember that altitude increases alcohol's blood glucose-lowering effect.

If you take rapid-acting insulin, wait until your food comes down the aisle before you inject. A delay in the meal service could spell trouble if you take your insulin prematurely. Stretch frequently, and occasionally walk briefly up and down the aisle to prevent muscle stiffness and increase your circulation. If you want to sleep, ask the flight attendant to wake you at mealtime or when you need to take your medication.

If You Travel by Rail or Bus

Unless they are major terminals, most rail or bus stations and train dining cars offer limited food choices you would do best to avoid. If you wish to eat in the waiting area or on board, it is safest to pack along your meal. Try to eat at whatever hour is your regular time, even if you are crossing a time zone. Check your blood glucose level frequently, and keep plenty of snacks handy in case there are delays. If you will be arriving at your destination in the late evening, do some advance research to learn whether a grocery or convenience store will be open in the area. If not, be sure to bring along enough food to tide you over until breakfast.

If You Drive

Check your blood glucose level frequently, and keep plenty of snacks handy in case you get tangled in a traffic jam, have car trouble, or become lost. If you feel any hypoglycemic symptoms, pull over and treat them using the 15 rule (see page 16) or as directed by your health-care team. Wait until your blood sugar level returns to your target range before resuming your travels.

Don't overdo it. Limit your driving time to twelve hours each day, and get adequate rest. Bring along meals you pack at home, or dine at or obtain takeaways from restaurants that can coordinate with your dietary needs; avoid settling for fast-food outlets. Try to maintain regular medication, snack, and meal times, and pull over every few hours to stretch your legs and help improve your circulation. If you bring insulin, don't place it in areas that become hot, such as the trunk or glove compartment. Instead, store it in a specially designed cool pack.

If You Hike, Camp, Ski, or Boat

It is lots of fun to spend time in the great outdoors. But don't do it alone. Always head out with a partner who knows that you have diabetes, and tell others where you are headed and when you plan to return. Use sunscreen and insect repellent, wear comfortable shoes that fit your activity, and protect your food supply from animals. Pack adequate supplies including a first aid kit, water, and fast-acting carbohydrate snacks You're obviously not going to be near anyplace where you can buy additional snacks, and help may be hours away if for some reason your return is delayed. So, if you use insulin, bring a Glucagon kit and review its use with your partner. This kit provides quick and effective emergency treatment if your glucose level drops to a dangerously low level. Ask your healthcare team to teach you how to use this kit properly.

If You Cruise

A luxury cruise is a treat. Physical activities are planned for you, medical experts are on call, entertainment is 'round the clock, and tempting meals are displayed for your eating pleasure. The big challenge is the buffet. Many cruise lines now offer lower-carb and low-calorie options, but it is up to you to choose the right items in the appropriate amounts. Request a sample menu ahead of time to decide which foods best fit into your meal plan, and ask if the chef is amenable to whipping up lower-carb variations of some of these items. Try the Plate Method of meal planning that was described in chapter 3, so that you can control your portion sizes.

Partake in the physical activity classes that are offered, take brisk walks around the deck, or go for a swim to compensate for any extra food that you may sample. The exercise that you do each day may help lower your blood glucose level for up to about 48 hours. And let the staff know that you have diabetes.

If you aren't ready to face a regular cruise, try a diabetes one. Many hospitals and organizations, such as the Joslin Diabetes Center in Boston, sponsor them throughout the year. Healthy foods are on the menu, the aerobic activities are plentiful, and educational lectures on topics such as menu planning, medication, exercise, glucose monitoring, and research are offered by expert teachers. Bob

Saltzberg, of Diabetesworkshopcruises.com, has planned diabetes cruises for more than seventeen years. His cruises travel to stunning locations including the Caribbean, Bermuda, and Alaska.

You can also participate in a diabetes conference that is held in beautiful surroundings. Childrenwithdiabetes.com holds annual conferences in Cancun, Mexico, and Orlando, Florida; and TCOYD.org runs conferences in several locations, including Hawaii and San Diego. The American Diabetes Association hosts educational seminars in different cities throughout the United States as well. Visit diabetes.org for information.

CHOOSE YOUR JUMP-START PLEDGE

- I pledge to assemble an emergency kit that I can bring along when I travel.
- I pledge to spend an hour this week, researching online the diabetic menus available on flights to a place I'd like to go.
- I pledge to book accommodations this week, for a short getaway to test my vacationing skills.
- I pledge to buy a thermal food container, thermos bottle, and cold packs this week, so that I can be ready to go whenever the travel big bites.
- I pledge to [your choice] for one week.

TAKE CHARGE

LET LIFE TAKE YOU WHERE YOU WANT TO GO!

10

SAY YES TO . . .
Changing the Future

I SEE MANY patients who ask, "Why me? Why did I have to get this disease?" Perhaps you've asked these same questions also. I wish I could tell you exactly why your life has taken this particular path, but I can't. What I can say is that having diabetes has given you a unique opportunity to understand the needs of others who have this disease. With that information, you can make a real difference. You may believe that you have little power, but that is not true. You can change the lives and the perceptions of people around you. Your actions can be as simple as a phone call or suggestion at your workplace, or as involved as planning a walkathon. Here are a few ways that you can help improve the world of diabetes:

IN THIS CHAPTER, YOU WILL:

- Discover how you can make a difference in the lives of others with diabetes.
- Learn how to become a diabetes advocate, contact legislators, and change our laws.

- Find out about how to participate in a research study.
- Evaluate how much power your financial gift can have.
- Learn how volunteering helps your health as much as it helps the lives of others.
- Make a Jump-Start Pledge that can change the future of diabetes.

It started with a single phone call after Hurricane Katrina hit the United States:

"This is Tom."
"Is this *dLife*?"
"Yes, sir."
"Turn on the news."
"Excuse me?"
"TURN ON THE NEWS."

A row of TV sets was right outside my office, so I ran to take a look. There, on a broken house somewhere in Louisiana, was a man lying on a rooftop next to two words painted in red: "Help" and "Diabetic."

I returned to the phone.

"What are you going to do about that?" the man asked.

I could still see the pictures on the screen. I wondered what would happen to my daughter Kaitlyn, who has diabetes, if Long Island were suddenly ripped at its seams from a natural disaster. Who would be there for her? At that moment, I knew that I had to act quickly.

"Sir, every ounce of energy I own and every resource we have will be given to these efforts. You have my word."

"Thank you...."
"Yes, sir..."
"... wait ... uh ... hey ..."
"Yes?"
"God bless you."

This call was answered by Tom Karlya, vice president and executive producer of *dLifeTV*, and launched one of the most impressive private medical support drives in history. The offices of *dLife* coordinated the distribution of millions of dollars worth of medicine, supplies, and support to individuals with diabetes who lived in areas that were devastated by the storm; countless lives were saved.

STEP 19

Find a Way to Make a Difference

LET YOUR VOICE BE HEARD

IF YOU HAVE diabetes, you probably have strong opinions about diabetes research, health care, and insurance that deserve to be heard. Help convince legislators to pass legislation that improves the lives of you and those around you. To do this, become an American Diabetes Association (ADA) diabetes advocate, at diabetes.org or 1–800-DIABETES. As an advocate, you will receive e-mail legislative updates, action requests, and guidance on how to accomplish each task. Here is the type of note that you might receive in your e-mail:

```
Dear Supporter of the American Diabetes
Association:
   The U.S. Senate will soon vote on a bill that
could leave millions of Americans with diabetes
without insurance coverage for their diabetes
needs. The bill, S. 1955, will preempt the 46
state laws, passed over the last decade with
bipartisan support, that require state-regu-
lated health plans to cover diabetes education,
equipment, and supplies. As American Diabetes
```

Association volunteers, this legislation directly impacts our mission. We must join together and stop it.

Today, the organization is asking for your help in our efforts to lobby senators and secure their opposition to S. 1955 in its current state, as it fails to protect state diabetes coverage regulations.

Things you can do to oppose S. 1955 include:

- Register with our Online Action Center. Once you register, you will see this issue under the heading "Preserve Diabetes Coverage Laws!"
  Click on that link and send an e-mail to your U.S. senators. Sample language is already prepared.
- Know your U.S. senators or one of their staffers personally, or interested in getting to know them? They are on recess this week, so schedule a meeting in the district office before March 27th to talk about why S. 1955 will harm people with diabetes. Use these talking points (click link) for meetings.
- Have five minutes to make a phone call? Phone calls can really have a big impact. With five minutes, you can call your senators' D.C. offices to urge a NO vote on undoing state-mandated health insurance coverage. Use these talking points (click link) for your phone call.

Become more familiar with S. 1955. Click here to access the S. 1955 Fact Sheet and more. Thank you for your commitment to the Association and your help in its mission: To prevent and cure diabetes, and to improve the lives of all people affected by diabetes.

Sincerely,
Lawrence T. Smith
Chair of the Board,
American Diabetes Association

As you can see, each note that you receive as a diabetes advocate provides instructions and details about an issue. You receive information links and talking points, and are guided every step of the way. You don't have to be an expert or have past political experience. If you don't know who your legislators are or how to contact them, the advocacy department can make this information available to you. Your help is needed, and you receive free training.

HELP OTHERS ACHIEVE THEIR RIGHTS

SADLY, MANY INDIVIDUALS with diabetes encounter discrimination at work and in school. If you know of students who are not getting their needs met, encourage them to visit the "Diabetes at School" section of childrenwithdiabetes.com. It contains information on students' legal rights and offers materials that explain diabetes and its treatment to teachers, roommates, and classmates. If you have friends with diabetes who experience discrimination at their workplace, report the incident to the ADA at diabetes.org or 1–800-DIABETES. Don't stay silent. You can direct people in need to information that will make a significant difference in their lives.

You can also make some noise about your own personal issues. In 2005, Congress repealed a blanket ban on insulin-treated individuals from driving commercial vehicles.

This change should have prevented Jeff Mather from losing his job as a truck driver, but it didn't. His boss obviously did not adhere to the law. Instead of bemoaning his situation and moving on, he chose to advocate on his own behalf:

> I am a truck driver who just recently developed diabetes. I never saw it coming. I lost 70 pounds in a single month. Little did I know that diabetes would rob me of my career as a truck driver. I thought at the time that I was one of my company's best employees. I did it well and enjoyed the opportunity to see this wonderful country. However, I was just a number and could be easily replaced.
>
> Recently, I began to speak out on behalf of other diabetic truckers who want to return to their jobs. I've been contacting the legislators in Washington, D.C. The American Diabetes Association provided me with lots of support, information, and guidance. My radio interview will air soon on NPR, about my fight to return to my career, and I have two articles coming out. One will be in *Roadstar*, a trucking newspaper, and the other in *The Trucker*.
>
> One of the other things I hope to do is ride a bike in the American Diabetes Association's annual Tour de Cure fundraiser. If I can help the ADA raise money, I am willing to do so. They have done so much for me. I want to give something back to them and prove to everyone that becoming diabetic it is not the end of your life; you can go on. If you want something badly enough it will happen . . . The company I worked for turned their back on me when I fell ill, and that hurt a lot. I promise that I will never turn my back on anyone in need and I will help the ADA with their quest to find a cure for this. I don't want anyone to have to go through what I have.

Jeff shared his story on the dLife.com and dearjanis.com message boards, and his efforts were noticed. His voice is now being heard and supported by great numbers of individuals.

BE PART OF THE CURE

WE ALL ACHE to find a cure for diabetes as quickly as possible. Help fund research projects or volunteer to be part of an actual research study. When Bill King participated in the landmark Diabetes Control and Complications Trial that was conducted from 1983 to 1993 by the National Institute of Diabetes and Digestive and Kidney Diseases, he received much more than he expected. This study showed that well-controlled blood glucose levels could slow the onset and development of diabetes-related eye, kidney, and nerve disease. As a participant in the study, Bill received counseling, free medication, excellent medical care, and a generous amount of education.

By the end of the study, Bill knew as much about diabetes as many experts. As a board member of the Diabetes Exercise and Sports Association, Bill speaks to many groups about ways to improve their health. Even though several years have passed, he continues to comment on his research experience when he gives these talks. It was a meaningful experience that not only improved his personal diabetes control, but altered his view of diabetes. He is now extremely positive about his future and the future of others who live with the disease. He gained an incredible amount from participating in that study, and encourages everyone to be part of ongoing research efforts. Ask your health-care provider about research projects in your area that are searching for volunteers, or visit clinicaltrials.com and find out about health-related studies in your state.

SEND A CHILD TO CAMP

FEW THINGS ARE as wonderful for a child with diabetes as a summer camp experience. They enjoy all of the normal activities of camp life, such as sports, swimming, and arts and crafts, but do it in an environment that is safe and supportive. They get to meet other children who, like them, wear insulin pumps, take injections, check their blood glucose, and count carbohydrates. Campers participate in self-esteem building experiences, and make friends with others kids their age who have the same worries and problems as they do. Best of all, they get to forget that they have diabetes and concern themselves with mundane, fun things, such as nature projects, winning races, and crafts. If you have a special place in your heart for children, donate a diabetes camp scholarship or volunteer at a diabetes camp. Your gift will provide a life-altering summer adventure to a deserving child. The youngster's parents will benefit as well. They will enjoy a worry-free summer, knowing that their child is having fun in a healthy and nurturing environment. Check out the extensive list of camps throughout the world at diabetescamps.org, the official site of the Diabetes Camping Association, or at childrenwithdiabetes.com.

Tiffany, a young teen with type 1 diabetes, has enjoyed attending her diabetes camp for eleven years:

> [Camp] has been a lifesaver for me. I developed a lot of independence and confidence with managing my diabetes. Sometimes it can be hard for kids who feel alone. It really is hard to make diabetes a part of your everyday life. Diabetes camp really helped me in that respect.

HELP RAISE FUNDS

HAVE YOU EVER participated in a diabetes walkathon or other fund-raising event? As you walk with hundreds of others, you make friends, get exercise, spread diabetes awareness, and raise funds for a great cause. The Juvenile Diabetes Research Foundation sponsors two hundred different walks each year, in which more than 500,000 people participate. They offer a carnival environment filled with entertainment, food, and fun. In 2004, diabetes walks raised $81 million for diabetes research.

Cycle by Proxy

If you prefer to let others do the "walking" for you, contact Phil and Joe. Phil Southerland, a graduate of the University of Georgia, and Charles "Joe" Eldridge, a graduate of Auburn University, are two young cyclists who recently formed a competitive cycling team known as TeamType1 that raises funds for research and for young people with diabetes who are denied health insurance.

Phil was diagnosed with type 1 diabetes at seven months old. It was so unusual for anyone to develop diabetes at such a young age that he had difficulty finding anyone to make the diagnosis. He had lost ten pounds and was told that he had the flu. His mom, however, continued to believe that he had a very serious problem and finally drove him to the emergency room of a major research hospital, where she was told that if she had waited one more day, he would have died. Today, Phil is a healthy, athletic cyclist who is passionate about helping others with diabetes. Joe was diagnosed with type 1 diabetes at the age of ten. He has always been active in a variety of different athletic activities and finally became hooked on competitive cycling at the age of twenty. In addition to their shared fund-raising goals, Joe's personal goal is to show other individuals with diabetes that they can compete at the highest level in any sport even if they have diabetes.

You and your friends pledge money per mile while Phil, Joe, and the rest of their team ride. TeamType1 recently broke all records when they came in first place in the annual Race Across America, a grueling eight-day competition. The team of eight, who all have diabetes, raced 3,052 miles across the United States. Learn more about this amazing group at www.teamtype1.org.

WRITE A CHECK

Your financial gift can help send diabetes supplies to those in need through Childrenwithdiabetes.com and Insulin for Life (insulinforlife.org). It can further important research, increase the accessibility of education, and launch improvements in diabetes care. Research organizations, educational groups, children's camps, and other worthy groups need funds to support their projects. Many of these organizations sell cards and gifts that you can send out from your business or family during the holiday season. Some offer credit cards, which send a small donation to the organization whenever you use it to make a purchase. Contact a group that you wish to support, and see what types of fund-raising opportunities they have available. Several worthwhile organizations include:

American Association of Diabetes Educators
(diabeteseducator.org)
American Diabetes Association
(diabetes.org or 1–800–DIABETES)
American Dietetic Association (eatright.org)
Childrenwithdiabetes.com
Diabetes Research Institute (diabetesresearch.org)
Joslin Diabetes Center (joslin.org)
Juvenile Diabetes Research Foundation (jdrf.org)
International Diabetes Federation (idf.org)
Taking Control of Your Diabetes (TCOYD.org)

INVEST YOUR FUNDS

If you use your savings to gain financially, it may not initially appear to have any humanitarian value. But it can. You have many choices for investing. If you place some of your funds in diabetes-related products and companies, you show support for items that you endorse, and encourage additional development to take place. David Kliff is the publisher of the *Diabetic Investor* newsletter, which reports on new and upcoming products in the ever-growing diabetes industry. He explains the current state of the diabetes business environment:

> If you break it down by market segments, obviously the biggest market is blood glucose monitoring. You have billions, absolutely billions of test strips sold each year. You have blood glucose monitoring that accounts for around $ 6 billion worldwide, you have the insulin market, which is about $4 billion dollars each year. Then you have all of the type 2 drugs, which is about $8 billion a year. So if you add those up, all of a sudden you have an $18 billion market, which most analysts expect to grow to over $30 billion just in a few short years.
>
> You have 20 million people in the United States who have diabetes . . . When you extrapolate that out to include the people who have prediabetes . . . you're talking about another 40 million people. So, this is an absolutely enormous market . . . You know, there is nothing wrong, from my perspective . . . from taking some of your hard-earned money and investing in the good companies that can help this disease get better.

When you support products that you like, it helps them remain on the market and encourages other companies to make similar items. As David mentioned above, a cure is the ultimate goal. But we don't have a cure coming down the pike in the near future, so the best we can hope for is the development of more and better diabetes products.

PARTICIPATE IN DIABETES EDUCATION AND OUTREACH

NONPROFIT ORGANIZATIONS NEED warm bodies, not just cash. Consider volunteering at a diabetes educational seminar. You don't need to be a speaker; they always need help with registration and other tasks, and by assisting with the programs and materials you will stay on the cutting edge of new information about diabetes. The American Diabetes Association hosts Diabetes Expos in many different communities and appreciates volunteer participation. Taking Control of Your Diabetes (TCOYD.org) sponsors conferences in numerous states, including Hawaii, and would welcome your efforts as well. Or check your local newspaper for support groups that could use a hand. If an organization was helpful to you, show your thanks by extending their hand to others. And your active volunteerism may have an additional benefit:

STEP 20
Enjoy the Benefits of Helping Others

MULTIPLE RESEARCH STUDIES show that individuals who volunteer on a regular basis have reduced levels of depression and significantly lower death rates than those who do not volunteer. Dr. David J. Demko, a gerontologist, developed the Original Death Calculator: Life Expectancy Quiz to help evaluate a person's life expectancy. While designing this quiz, which is posted at www.demko.com he discovered that people who participated in some type of volunteer activity each day added two years to their life.

Dr. Demko does not believe that long life is the result of "smart genes and dumb luck." Eighty percent of longevity is based on the lifestyle that you choose to lead. According to current research, living to the age of 100 depends on five factors:

- The genes that you've inherited, which give you a good start in life
- Your personal outlook, as a life filled with meaning lasts longer
- The food choices you make

- Your physical activity level
- Your mental health

What you do to help others is your decision alone. Diabetes can be challenging. If you are living well with this condition, reach out to others and help them along. If you have no time to lick stamps, make phone calls, or participate in a walkathon, you can still make a difference. Don't underestimate the power that you have. You can change the future.

CHOOSE YOUR JUMP-START PLEDGE

- I pledge to sign up as an ADA diabetes advocate and participate in one of their activities this week.
- I pledge to learn about one of the organizations listed in this chapter, and send in a donation of support this week.
- I pledge to sign up for an hour's worth of volunteer work this week.
- I pledge to [your choice] for one week.

TAKE CHARGE

HELP SUPPORT IMPROVEMENTS IN THE WORLD OF DIABETES.

Afterword

> I did it my way.
> —*Frank Sinatra*

I HOPE THAT I've helped you discover how to live with diabetes on your *own* terms—to take care of your diabetes in a way that feels right to you, reach out to experts you respect, and determine if a particular approach works for you. I hope that you are now inspired to take an active role in determining the type of care that you receive, feel more confident to make healthier food choices, and are ready to do activities that you enjoy.

Take out the list of actions that you've decided to try while reading this book. Make an appointment to discuss these new actions with your health-care team and see if they are appropriate for you then make them into easy-to-implement Jump-Start Pledges. Choose one to start with, and you'll be on your way. I'd love to hear what goals you've chosen for yourself. Please share them with me at www.dearjanis.com. Those who are close to you may be surprised by the new you. As your friends see the new joy that you have in your life, hopefully they will applaud you for your ability to embrace and enjoy a full and exciting life with diabetes. Good luck with all that you do. Remember, when you live on your own terms, your life is truly your own.

JANIS ROSZLER, RD, CDE, LD/N

Selected References

Abela, G. S., and K. Aziz. 2005. Cholesterol crystals cause mechanical damage to biological membranes: a proposed mechanism of plaque rupture and erosion leading to arterial thrombosis. *Clinical Cardiology* 28:413–20.

Allen, K, B. Shykoff, J. Izzo, Jr. 2001. Pet ownership, but not ACE inhibitor therapy, blunts home blood pressure responses to mental stress. *Hypertension* 38:815.

American Diabetes Association. 2006. *Clinical Practice Recommendations.* Diabetes Care 29 (Suppl 1): S10–11.

Colberg, Sheri. 2006. *The 7-Step Diabetes Fitness Plan.* New York: Marlowe & Company.

Covington, M. 2001. Traditional Chinese medicine in the treatment of diabetes. *Diabetes spectrum* 14:154–59.

Ezzo, J, T. Donner, D. Nickols, and M. Cox. 2001. Is massage useful in the management of diabetes? A systematic Review. *Diabetes Spectrum* 14:218–24.

Garrow D, and L. Egede. 2006. Association between complementary and alternative medicine use, preventive care practices, and use of conventional medical services among adults with diabetes. *Diabetes Care.* 29:15–19.

Gehling E. 2001. The next step: depression. *Newsflash.* Publication of Diabetes Care and Education, a Dietetic Practice Group of the American Dietetic Association, 22(5).

Hernandez-Ruiz, E. 2005. Effect of music therapy on the anxiety levels and sleep patterns of abused women in shelters. *Journal of Music Therapy.* Summer, 42(2):140–58.

Hooper, P. L. 1999. Hot-tub therapy for type 2 diabetes mellitus. *New England Journal of Medicine* 341(12) (September 16): 924–5.

King, D. E, A. G, Mainous, III, and W. S. Pearson. 2002. C-reactive protein, diabetes and attendance at religious services. *Diabetes Care* 25:1172–76.

Lee, H. R. 2003. Effects of relaxing music on stress response of patients with acute myocardial infarction. (article in Korean) *Taehan Kanho Hakhoe Chi* 33(6) (October): 693–704.

Lee, S, R. Hudson, K. Kilpatrick, et al. 2005. Caffeine ingestion is associated with reductions in glucose uptake independent of obesity and type 2 diabetes before and after exercise training. *Diabetes Care* 28:566–72.

Lloyd, C., J. Smith, K. Weinger, 2005. K. Stress and diabetes: A review of the links. *Diabetes Spectrum* 18:121–27.

Nilsson U., M. Unosson, and N. Rawal. 2005. Stress reduction and analgesia in patients exposed to calming music postoperatively: a randomized controlled trial. *European Journal of Anaesthesiology* 22(2) (February): 96–102.

____. *PDR for Nutritional Supplements.* 2001. Montvale, NJ: Thomson PDR.

Polonsky, William H. *Diabetes Burnout.* 1999. Alexandria, VA: American Diabetes Association.

Rice, B. I. 2001. Mind-body Interventions. *Diabetes spectrum* 14:213–17

Roszler, J. 2005. Appendix C: Use of herbs, supplements, and alternative therapies. *American Dietetic Association Guide to Diabetes Medical Nutrition Therapy and Education.* Chicago, American Dietetic Association.

Samuel-Hodge, C. D., S. W. Headen, A. H. Skelly, et al. 2000. Influences on day-to-day self-management of type 2 diabetes among African-American women. Spirituality, the multi-caregiver role, and other social context factors. *Diabetes Care* 23:928–33.

Recommended Books and Web Sites

Books

Anderson, Bob, and Martha Funnell. *The Art of Empowerment. Stories and Strategies for Diabetes Educators*. Alexandria, VA: American Diabetes Association, 2000.

Becker, Gretchen. *The First Year: Type 2 Diabetes: An Essential Guide for the Newly Diagnosed, 2nd edition*. New York: Marlowe & Company, 2007.

Duke, James A. *The Green Pharmacy Herbal Handbook*. New York: Rodale Reach, 2000.

Edelman, Steven, V. *Taking Control of Your Diabetes*. Caddo, OK: Professional Communications, Inc., 2001.

Polonsky, William H. *Diabetes Burnout, What to Do When You Can't Take It Anymore*. Alexandria, VA: American Diabetes Association, 1999.

Rubin, Alan L. *Diabetes for Dummies*, 2nd ed. Indiannapolis: Wiley Publishing, 2004.

Roszler, Janis, William H. Polonsky, and Steven V. Edelman. *The Secrets of Living and Loving with Diabetes*. Chicago: Surrey Books, 2004.

Warshaw, Hope, and Karmeen Kulkarni. *Complete Guide to Carb Counting*, 2nd ed. Alexandria, VA: American Diabetes Association, 2004.

Wolpert, Howard. *Smart Pumping for People with Diabetes*. Alexandria, VA: American Diabetes Association, 2002.

Web Sites

aace.com—The official Web site of the American Association of Clinical Endocrinologists

americanheart.org—The official Web site of the American Heart Association angelarose.com/famousdiabetics—This Web site lists famous people with diabetes

caloriecontrol.org—The official Web site of the Calorie Control Council. Offers information about sweeteners and other weight-loss products

calorieking.com—This Web site offers nutrient information

cartoonmd.com—This Web site, created by endocrinologist Justin Grady Matrisciano, uses cartoons and animated videos to explain the action of diabetes medications and other diabetes-related concepts

centerwatch.com—This Web site lists medical research studies that are seeking volunteers

childrenwithdiabetes.com—This Web site provides support and information for individuals of all ages with diabetes and their families.

consumerlab.com—An independent Web site that reviews the safety and effectiveness of herbs and supplements

dearjanis.com—My personal Web site—contains an interactive message board, articles, podcasts and radio show interviews

diabetes.org—The official Web site of the American Diabetes Association

diabetescamps.org—Lists diabetes summer camps for children and offers ways to support these terrific programs

diabeteseducator.org—The official Web site of the American Association of Diabetes Educators. Offers an educator locator service

diabetes.niddk.nih.gov—This is the Web site of the National Diabetes Information Clearinghouse, run by the National Institute of Diabetes and Digestive and Kidney Diseases and National Institutes of Health (NIH)

Diabetes-exercise.org—The official Web site of DESA, the Diabetes Exercise and Sports Association

diabetesworkshopcruises.com—A Web site that highlights available vacation cruises

dLife.com—The Web site affiliated with the *dLifeTV* weekly television program on CNBC

drinet.org—Official Web site of the Diabetes Research Institute

eatright.org—The official Web site of the American Dietetic Association

ediets.com/nt—eDiets.com's free Nutrition Tracker tool

foodpsychology.cornell.edu—Web site of the Cornell University Food and Brand Lab

healthfinder.gov—Run by the U.S. Department of Health and Human Services, this Web site provides a list of reliable Web sites

idf.org—Official Web site of the International Diabetes Federation insulinforlife.org—An organization that sends insulin to those in need throughout the world

intellihealth.com—Consumer medical information from Harvard Medical School

jdrf.org—The official Web site of the Juvenile Diabetes Research Foundation

joslin.org—The official Web site of the Joslin Diabetes Center in Boston

medlineplus.gov—This Web site provides information about medications and medical conditions. Sponsored by the U.S. National Library of Medicine and NIH

mendosa.com/diabetes.htm—An extensive diabetes directory

michelnischan.com—The official Web site of Chef Michel Nischan

nhlbi.nih.gov/chd/lifestyles.htm—Web site of the Therapeutic Lifestyle Changes section of the National Heart, Lung, and Blood Institute (NHLBI)

nwcr.ws—Web site of the National Weight Control Registry

platemethod.com—The Web site of the Idaho Plate Method diabetes meal planning tool

quackwatch.com—Provides a guide to medical misinformation and health fraud; check out health-related Internet rumors at this Web site

snopes.com—Debunks Internet rumors of all types

teamtype1.org—The official Web site of the fundraising cycling team headed by Phil Southerland and Joe Eldridge

TCOYD.org—The Web site for Taking Control of Your Diabetes, an educational organization founded by Dr. Steven V. Edelman

urbanlegends.about.com—An additional Web site that debunks Internet rumors

webmd.com—A reliable source of medical information

Acknowledgments

I AM DEEPLY indebted to Howard Steinberg and Paula Ford-Martin of *dLifeTV* for generously allowing me to share dLife.com podcasts throughout this book, and to all of the experts and individuals who contributed their wisdom and experiences. I am especially grateful to my publisher, Matthew Lore; and my husband Myer; and children Elisheua, Shira, Rachel, and Amichai; for their enthusiastic support.

Index

A

A1C test
  blood glucose range, 8–10
  overview, 3–5, 52
  timing of, 11–15, 120–21, 123, 158
AADE-7(tm) Self-Care Behaviors worksheet, 99–100
A-B-C tool
  blood pressure, 5–6, 36–38, 72, 133
  goal setting for, 43
  See also A1C test; cholesterol and other lipids
abnormal glucose level corrections, 15–19, 43
acanthosis nigricans, 82
ACE inhibitors, 36
acesulfame K, 110
Actos (pioglitazone), 32
acupressure, 79
acupuncture, 79–80
ADA. *See* American Diabetes Association
adapting to change
  choosing acceptance, 165
  in glucose levels, 10–11
  recipe adjustments, 107–9, 110–15, 116
  wearing an insulin pump, 28–29

advocacy, 167–70
air travel, 159–61
ALA (alpha-lipoic acid), 39, 79
alcohol, 74, 122–23
allicin, 73
alopecia, 82
alpha-glucosidase inhibitors, 31
alpha-lipoic acid (ALA), 39, 79
Amaryl (glimepiride), 31
American Association of Clinical Endocrinologists, 9, 98
American Association of Diabetes Educators, 94, 99–100
American Diabetes Association (ADA)
  advertising review panel, 87
  blood glucose level recommendation, 9
  diabetes advocates, 167–70
  Diabetes Expos, 176
  on diuretics, 36
  on glycemic index, 62
  on grams of carbohydrate per day, 55–56
  recommendations for fat intake, 72
American Dietetic Association, 150
American Dietetic Association Guide to Diabetes Medical Nutrition Therapy and Education (ADA), 39–41
American Heart Association, 72
amputations, avoiding, 80–82

Anderson, Bob, 96
angiotensin receptor blockers (ARBs), 36
anodyne therapy, 79
Apidra (insulin glulisine), 17–19, 25
ARBs (angiotensin receptor blockers), 36
aromatherapy, 143
artificial sweeteners, 110–12
aspartame, 111
aspirin, 36–37, 71
autonomic nerves, 77–78
Avandia (rosiglitazone), 32

B

background retinopathy, 75–76
basal rate, 27
BC-ADM (board-certified advanced diabetes manager), 94–95
bilberry, 76
biofeedback training, 79
bitter melon, 34
blood glucose levels
    alcohol and, 74, 122–23
    damage from excess glucose, 68, 83
    for driving, 14–15
    insulin pump and, 24–31
    maintenance techniques, 15–19, 43
    target range, 8–11
    testing, 11–15, 120–21, 123, 158
    See also hypoglycemia; insulin; medication choices
blood lipids. *See* cholesterol and other lipids
blood pressure, 5–6, 36–38, 72, 133
blood sugar highs with insulin pump, 29
blood vessels. *See* cardiovascular disease
BMI (body mass index), 47–50
boating, 162–63
bolus, 27, 30
books on diabetes, 93, 187
Brackenridge, Betty, xv, 126–27, 139
Brand-Miller, Jennie, 62
Brink, Stuart, xv, 122
Brown, J. Anthony, xv, 140–41

bus, traveling via, 162
business meetings and events, 120–23
Byetta, 33

C

caffeine, 74, 142
Cairns, Douglas, xv, 154–56
calcium channel blockers, 36
calorieking.com, 60
camping, 162–63
capsaicin topical cream, 79
carbohydrates, 13, 27–28, 31, 55–62, 73–74
cardiovascular disease
    avoiding, 39–41, 70–74
    causes of, 69–70
    hypertension, 5–6, 36–38, 72, 133
    See also cholesterol and other lipids
Carpentier, Fran, xvi, 88–89
certified diabetes educators (CDEs), 52, 94–95, 139–40
change. *See* adapting to change
Chicken Florentine, 107–9
children, 109–10, 123, 169, 171–72, 174
childrenwithdiabetes.com, 123, 164, 169, 172, 174
Chinese medicine, 79–80
choices, value of having, xiv
cholesterol and other lipids
    fat intake and, 72, 112–13
    limiting intake of, 71–74
    overview, 6–7, 8
    treatment options, 38–41
    xanthelasmas from imbalance, 83
chromium, 34
cinnamon, 34, 39
coenzyme Q10, 35
coffee, 74, 142
complementary options to medication, 33–35
complication avoidance
    eye care, 75–76
    foot care, 80–82

Index

heart and blood vessel care, 69–74
kidney care, 76–77
mouth and gum care, 83–85
nervous system care, 77–80
overview, 67–69, 85
research on, 171
skin care, 82–83
complications
  from A1C level over 7%, 4, 9
  from depression, 150
  from high blood pressure, 5, 6
  from high LDL cholesterol, 7
  overview, 67–68
  sexual, 78, 132–35
  from supplements, 34, 40, 73
conferences, 164
consumerlab.com, 34, 71, 73
credentials of information resources, 93, 94–95
cruise ships, 163

D

Dare to Dream (Cairns), 156
dating, 130–32
Davidson, Paul C., 18
dawn phenomenon, 14
dearjanis.com, 21, 63, 92
dehydration, 82, 83
dental appointments, 84–85
depression treatments, 149–51
DHA and EPA (fish oils), 40
diabetes, type 1 versus type 2, 127
diabetes advocacy, 167–70
diabetes conferences, 164
Diabetes Control and Complications Trial, 171
diabetes cruises, 163–64
diabeteseducator.org, 99, 100
Diabetes Expos, 176
Diabetes Myths, Misconceptions, and Big Fat Lies (Brackenridge, et al.), 126–27, 139
diet choices
  alcohol, 74, 122–23
  cholesterol and, 71–74

family complaints about, 109–10
fats, 72, 112–13
fish, 70–71
marketing and, 104–6
overview, 103–4, 107, 117
recipe adjustments, 107–9, 110–15, 116
shopping wisely, 115–16
snacks, 121, 156
sodium intake, 37–38, 77, 113–14
weight maintenance, 64
See also meal-planning method choices; supplements
dietetic versus diabetic foods, 116
dietitians, 52, 55, 61, 94, 140
diuretics, 36
dLifeTV (CNBC), 93
Drago, Lorena, xvi, 61
driving with diabetes, 14–15, 162
dry mouth, 85

E

Edelman, Steven V., xvi, 32
ED (erectile dysfunction), 69, 132–34
eDiets.com, 60
education programs, 175–76
eggs, 71
1,800 rule, 18–19
Eldridge, Charles "Joe," 173
empowerment approach to diabetes care, 96–101
endocrinologists, 9, 98
endorphins, 41
Eng, John, 33
Enova oil, 113
EPA and DHA (fish oils), 40, 70–71
Equal, 111
erectile dysfunction (ED), 69, 132–34
evaluating where you're at, 2–8, 104–6
evening primrose oil, 40, 79
exchange list sample, 56–57
exenatide, 33
exercise
  benefits of, 133, 142
  as "magic pill," 41–44

testing before, during, and after, 14
types of, 116, 144–45, 162–63
eye care, 75–76

F

family complaints about diet choices, 109–10
family gatherings, 123–27
fats, 72, 112–13. *See also* cholesterol and other lipids
FDA, 110–11
feet, caring for, 80–82
fenugreek, 35, 40
fiber, 59, 114
fibrates, 39
15/15 rule, 16–17
first aid kits, 157
fish oils, 40, 70–71
food choices. *See* diet choices
food on hand, 121, 156
food shopping, 115–16
foot care, 80–82
Forbidden Foods Diabetic Cooking (Powers), 106
foreign countries, traveling in, 156–57, 160–61
Foster-Powell, Kaye, 62
Freeman, Kris, xiii
friends, 63, 127–30, 149
fundraising, 172–73
fungal infections, 82, 84
Funnell, Martha, 96–97

G

gamma linolenic acid (GLA), 40
garlic, 40, 73
Gemfibrozil, 39
Gila monsters, 33
ginseng, 34
Glucagon kits, 163
glucose levels. *See* blood glucose levels
glucose meters, personal, 11–15, 120–21
Glucotrol (glipizide), 31
glycated hemoglobin, 4

glycemic index method for meal-planning, 62–64
Glyset (miglitol), 31
goal setting
    ABC goals, 43
    blood glucose levels, 8–11
    for exercise, 42–43
    postmeal goals, 9–11, 12–13, 17
    preparation for, 2–8
    weight goal, 46–47
    worksheet for, 99–100
Gorman, Christine, xvi, 89–90
Gottlieb, Sheldon, xvi, 69–70
guidance choices
    credentials to look for, 93, 94–95
    overview, 87–88, 101
    print media, 88–90, 93, 187
    for starting insulin, 26
    television programs, 93–94
    See also healthcare team; Internet resources
guilt avoidance, 1–8, 103
gum diseases, 83–85
gymnema sylvestre, 35

H

hair loss, 82
HDL cholesterol, 7–8, 39, 69, 72
healthcare team
    dietitians, 52, 55, 61, 94, 140
    insulin trainer, 9–10
    partnership with, 95–101
    preparing for visits, 100
    supplements, herbs, and, 34
heart. *See* cardiovascular disease
hemoglobin, glycated, 4
herbs and spices for salt replacement, 37–38
herbs and supplements, 33–35, 39–41, 76. *See also* supplements
high-density lipoproteins (HDL), 7–8, 39, 69, 72
hiking, 162–63
Hill, James O., 64

HMG-CoA reductase enzyme, 38
home glucose meters, 11–15, 120–21
hormones, 32–33, 36
Hostetter, Thomas, xvi, 76
hot peppers, 73
Humalog (insulin lispro), 17–19, 25
Hurricane Katrina, 166–67
hydrogenation, 7–8, 71
hypertension, 5–6, 36–38, 72, 133
hypnosis, 79
hypoglycemia
    avoiding, 16
    beta blockers and, 36
    causes of, 34, 39, 43, 122, 130–31, 132
    while driving, 162

I

Idaho Diabetes Care and Education practice group, 53
Idaho plate method for meal-planning, 53–55
identification, wearing, 123, 157
infomercials, 94
information. *See* guidance choices
insoluble fiber, 114
insulin
    carb counting and, 59–62
    correcting, 17–19
    overview, 25–31
    traveling with, 156–57
insulinforlife.org, 174
insulin pens, 30, 156–57, 159–60
insulin pump models, 31
insulin pumps, 24–31
insulin trainers, 9–10
Internet resources
    childrenwithdiabetes.com, 123, 164, 169, 172, 174
    consumerlab.com, 34, 71, 73
    dearjanis.com, 21, 63, 92, 183
    diabeteseducator.org, 99, 100
    diet information, 60, 63, 64
    fundraisers for uninsured diabetics, 173

Lifestyle Changes site, 72
    lists of, 91–92
    message boards and chat rooms, 63, 92
    overview, 90–92
    students' rights information, 169
    warning about, 14
intimacy issues, 78, 132–35
investing in diabetes-related companies, 174–75

J

Johns Hopkins University, 73–74
Joslin Diabetes Center (Boston), 163–64
Jump-Start Pledges, 1, 19–21, 146–49, 183
Juvenile Diabetes Research Foundation, 172–73

K

Karlya, Tom, 166–67
kidney care, 76–77
King, Bill, 171
Kliff, David, xvi, 175

L

Lantus (insulin glargine), 25
LDL cholesterol, 7, 69, 72, 74
lipids. *See* cholesterol and other lipids
long-acting insulin, 25
longevity and lifestyle, 180
low-density lipoproteins (LDL), 7, 69, 72, 74
Low GI Diet Revolution (Brand-Miller, et. al), 62

M

magazines, 89–90
magnesium, 40
marketing and food desires, 104–6
marketing effect on food choices, 104–6
massage, 144
Mather, Jeff, 169–70
McMillan-Price, Joanna, 62

meal-planning method choices
    carbohydrate-counting method, 55–62
    glycemic index method, 62–64
    for healthy cholesterol levels, 73–74
    Idaho plate method, 53–55
    lowering blood-sugar-raising effects, 114–15
    overview, 45–50, 62–63
    See also diet choices
medical identification, 123, 157
Medical University of South Carolina study, 146
medication choices
    blood sugar control, 13, 31–35
    complementary options to, 33–35
    for high blood pressure, 36–37
    for high cholesterol, 38–39
    overview, 23–25, 44
    for sexual complications, 133
    See also insulin
meditation, 145
medlineplus.gov, 34
meglitinides, 31
Menninger, Laura, xvi, 11–12
men's intimacy issues, 69, 78, 132–34
Metformin, 31, 33, 39
monitors, glucose, 11–15, 120–21
monounsaturated fatty acids, 72
Mother Love, xvi, 109–10
mouth and gum care, 83–85

N

National Cholesterol Education Program, 72
National Institute of Diabetes and Digestive and Kidney Diseases, 171
National Weight Control Registry (NWCR), 64
necrobiosis lipoidica diabeticorum, 82
nephropathy, 76
nervous system care, 77–80

neuropathy, 77–80, 82
newspapers, 88–89
niacin, 39
nicotine, damage from, 69–70, 142
nicotinic acid, 39
Novolog (insulin aspart), 17–19, 25
NutraSweet, 111
nutritionists, 95
nutrition label reading, 58–59
nwcr.ws, 64

O

office events, 120–23
omega-3 fatty acids, 70–71
oral medications, 31–32
Original Death Calculator, 176–80
outreach programs, 175–76

P

pancreas, imitating action of, 60
participation choices
    diabetes advocacy, 167–70
    funding options, 171–72, 174
    fundraising, 172–73
    investing intentionally, 174–75
    overview, 165–67
partners and pets, 149
party, hosting a, 127–30
pedometers, 116
penylketonuria (PKU), 111
peripheral nerves, 77–78
pets, value of, 149
pharmaceuticals. *See* medication choices
phenylalanine metabolization, 111
phenylethylamine (PEA), 41
polyunsaturated fats, 72
postmeal goals, 9–11, 12–13, 17
Powers, Maggie, 106
Prandin (repaglinide), 31
prayer power, 146
Precose (acarbose), 31
prioritizing, 100
proliferative retinopathy, 75–76
Prospective Diabetes Study, U.K., 6

protein intake, 76–77
pruritus, 83
psyllium, 35, 40
pump models, 31
pumps, 24–31

R

Race Across America, 173
rail, traveling via, 162
rapid-acting insulin, 17–19, 25, 59–62
realistic expectations, 139–40
recipe adjustments, 107–9, 110–15, 116
red blood cell life span, 4
relaxation techniques, 144–45
religious practices, 146
research, funding, 171
rest and sleep, 139–42
restaurants, dining in, 52, 121, 129–30, 162
retinopathy, 75–76
Rice, Donna, xvi, 78
Rubens, Peter Paul, 45
Rush University Medical Center (Chicago), 41–42

S

saccharin, 110–11
salt intake, 37–38, 77, 113–14
Saltzberg, Bob, 164
saturated fat, 71
Self-Care Behaviors worksheet, AADE-7(tm), 99–100
sexual complications, 78, 132–35
shoes and foot care, 81
shopping wisely, 115–16
60 Minutes, 93
skiing, 162–63
skin care, 82–83
sleep, value of, 140–42
smoking, damage from, 69–70, 142
snacks, 121, 156
social life choices
    dating, 130–32
    family gatherings, 123–27
    intimacy issues, 78, 132–35
    office events, 120–23
    overview, 119–20, 135–36
    parties with friends, 127–30
sodium intake, 37–38, 77, 113–14
soluble fiber, 114
Southerland, Phil, 173
spiritually-oriented practices, 146
Splenda, 111–12
Starlix (nateglinide), 31
statins, 38
Steinberg, Howard, 104
stevia, 112
stress avoidance choices
    depression treatments, 149–51
    exercise, 142
    overview, 137–40, 151
    partners and pets, 149
    relaxation techniques, 144–45
    religious practices, 146
    rest and sleep, 139–42
    water and/or aromatherapy, 143
students' rights, 169
sucralose, 111–12
sugar alcohols, 58–59
sugar grams in prepared foods, 58
Sugar Twin, 110–11
sulfonylureas, 13, 31, 33
Sundar "Sunny," 147–49
Sunette, 110
supplements
    as complement to medications, 33–35
    for eye health, 76
    garlic, 40, 73
    for heart health, 39–41
    for neuropathy, 78–79
    omega-3 fatty acids, 70–71
surgery, avoiding complications to, 34, 40, 73
sweeteners, artificial, 110–12
Sweet 'N Low, 110–11
Sweet One, 110
Symlin, 32

T

Taking Control of Your Diabetes, 32, 176
TeamType1, 173
television programs, 93–94
thiazolidinediones, 32
thrush, 84
Tour de Cure diabetes fundraiser, 170
trans fats, 7–8, 71
Trattner, Elizabeth, 142
travel choices
    advance preparation, 159–64
    expecting the unexpected, 157–58
    overview, 153–57, 164
treatments. *See* medication choices; supplements
triglycerides, 7–8, 38–39, 70–71
20/20, 93
type 1 versus type 2 diabetes, 127

U

United Kingdom Prospective Diabetes Study, 6
urinary infections, 134–35

V

vaginal infections, 134–35
vanadium, 35
vitamins C and E, 41
vitiligo, 83

W

Wansick, Brian, 104–6
Wasserman, Daniel, xvi, 79–80
water therapy, 143
weight, making realistic choices
    BMI, 47–49
    keeping weight off, 64
    overview, 45–46, 65
    plan of action choices, 50–52
    weight goal, 46–47
    See also meal-planning method choices
wine, 74
Wing, Rena, 64
women's intimacy issues, 78, 134–35

X

xanthelasmas, 83

Y

Yarus, Nina, xvi, 145
yeast infections, 134–35
yoga, 144–45

The Marlowe Diabetes Library
Good control is in your hands.

MARLOWE DIABETES LIBRARY titles are available from on-line and bricks-and-mortar retailers nationally. For more information about the Marlowe Diabetes Library or any of our books or authors, visit www.marlowepub.com/diabeteslibrary or e-mail us at goodcontrol@avalonpub.com

THE FIRST YEAR®—TYPE 2 DIABETES
An Essential Guide for the Newly Diagnosed, 2nd edition
Gretchen Becker | Foreword by Allison B. Goldfine, MD ■ $16.95

PREDIABETES
What You Need to Know to Keep Diabetes Away
Gretchen Becker | Foreword by Allison B. Goldfine, MD ■ $14.95

THE NEW GLUCOSE DIABETES REVOLUTION
The Definitive Guide to Managing Diabetes and Prediabetes Using the Glycemic Index
Dr. Jennie Brand-Miller, Kaye Foster-Powell, Dr. Stephen Colagiuri, Alan Barclay ■ $16.95
(Coming Spring 2007)

THE NEW GLUCOSE DIABETES REVOLUTION LOW GI GUIDE TO DIABETES
The Quick Reference Guide to Managing Diabetes Using the Glycemic Index
Dr. Jennie Brand-Miller and Kaye Foster-Powell with Johanna Burani ■ $6.95

THE 7 STEP DIABETES FITNESS PLAN
Living Well and Being Fit with Diabetes, No Matter Your Weight
Sheri R. Colberg, PhD | Foreword by Anne Peters, MD ■ $15.95

EATING FOR DIABETES
A Handbook and Cookbook—with More than 125 Delicious, Nutritious Recipes to Keep You Feeling Great and Your Blood Glucose in Check
Jane Frank ■ $15.95

TYPE 1 DIABETES
A Guide for Children, Adolescents, Young Adults—and Their Caregivers
Ragnar Hanas, MD, PhD | Forewords by Stuart Brink, MD, and Jeff Hitchcock ■ $24.95

KNOW YOUR NUMBERS, OUTLIVE YOUR DIABETES
Five Essential Health Factors You Can Master to Enjoy a Long and Healthy Life
Richard A. Jackson, MD, and Amy Tenderich ■ $14.95

INSULIN PUMP THERAPY DEMYSTIFIED
An Essential Guide for Everyone Pumping Insulin
Gabrielle Kaplan-Mayer | Foreword by Gary Scheiner, MS, CDE ■ $15.95

1,001 TIPS FOR LIVING WELL WITH DIABETES
Firsthand Advice that Really Works
Judith H. McQuown | Foreword by Harry Gruenspan, MD, PhD $16.95

DIABETES ON YOUR OWN TERMS
Janis Roszler, RD, CDE, LD/N ■ $14.95

THINK LIKE A PANCREAS
A Practical Guide to Managing Diabetes with Insulin
Gary Scheiner, MS, CDE | Foreword by Barry Goldstein, MD ■ $15.95

THE ULTIMATE GUIDE TO ACCURATE CARB COUNTING
Gary Scheiner, MS, CDE ■ $9.95

THE MIND-BODY DIABETES REVOLUTION
A Proven New Program for Better Blood Sugar Control
Richard S. Surwit, PhD, with Alisa Bauman ■ $14.95